Sperm in Shape

Sperm in Shape

A Guide to Male Reproductive Wellness

William Harper

Title: Sperm in Shape
Subtitle: A Guide to Male Reproductive Wellness
Author: William Harper

ISBN 9798300879990

Edition I, Ostrava, 2024

Introduction

Male reproductive health is a topic that still rarely takes center stage in open conversations. Much attention is given to women's fertility and health, while male fertility and sperm quality often remain in the background. Yet sperm quality is not just about the ability to have children—it is also a reflection of a man's overall health. Modern lifestyles, the increasing pace of work, environmental pollution, and poor dietary habits contribute to a decline in sperm quality for many men. This issue is becoming more widespread and affects men of all ages, regardless of their location or social status.

The purpose of this book is to change that narrative. We aim to highlight the critical role that daily choices play in reproductive health —from diet and physical activity to lifestyle and stress management. While many factors affecting sperm quality may seem beyond our control, there are countless areas where we can take deliberate and effective action.

This book provides a comprehensive guide to improving sperm quality and reproductive health. It focuses on scientifically proven methods and practical advice that can be easily implemented in daily life. We'll delve into the biological mechanisms that influence sperm production, as well as external factors such as environment, diet, and supplementation. Each chapter is designed to offer not only knowledge but also actionable tools for making positive changes.

This book is for all men—those planning fatherhood and those who simply want to invest in their health and longevity. Whether you're just beginning your journey toward better health or looking for ways to enhance your current situation, you'll find valuable insights and inspiration here to help you reach your goals.

Working on reproductive health is a process that requires consistency and commitment, but it also yields significant benefits. Improving sperm quality not only increases your chances of fatherhood but also enhances energy levels, overall well-being, and everyday quality of life. This book is your guide—a resource to help you understand what you can do to improve your health and enjoy the rewards.

I invite you to read on and hope that this journey will mark the beginning of positive changes in your life.

Why is it important to care about sperm quality?

Sperm quality is a topic that rarely comes up in everyday conversations, yet it is a crucial indicator of men's reproductive health. Modern lifestyles, increasing environmental pollution, stress, and unhealthy dietary habits are causing more and more men to face declining sperm quality. But why should you focus on this aspect of health and take conscious steps to improve it? The answer is simple: healthy sperm not only increase your chances of fatherhood but also contribute to better overall health, well-being, and resilience to the challenges of modern life.

The first reason to care about sperm quality is its direct impact on fertility. Sperm cells are the primary carriers of a man's genetic material, and their count, motility, and morphology determine the success of fertilization. Male fertility issues are becoming increasingly common—affecting approximately 40–50% of couples experiencing difficulty conceiving. In many cases, the underlying cause is related to sperm quality, which can often be improved through lifestyle changes, diet adjustments, and proper supplementation.

However, sperm quality is not just about fertility. It is also a reflection of a man's overall health. Hormonal imbalances, obesity, lack of physical activity, or chronic stress often manifest in reduced sperm quality. It's important to understand that reproductive health is an integral part of overall well-being. Improving sperm quality often coincides with better energy levels, enhanced mood, and greater resistance to illnesses.

Moreover, sperm quality is linked to the aging process. Maintaining healthy sperm can support longevity and delay the onset of age-related diseases. Free radicals, one of the main contributors to cellular aging, negatively impact sperm cells as well. Consuming antioxidants regularly and focusing on recovery through sleep and physical activity are actions that benefit both sperm quality and overall physical condition.

Caring for sperm quality also has psychological and emotional dimensions. Fertility issues can be a source of stress, frustration, and even a diminished sense of self-worth. Knowing that you are taking steps to improve your health can provide relief and a sense of control over the situation. Furthermore, reproductive health is important in the context of relationships. Open discussions about health and mutual efforts can strengthen bonds and build trust between partners.

Education also plays a significant role. Understanding the factors that affect sperm quality and how to improve them is an investment in the future. With this knowledge, men can make informed decisions about their lifestyle, diet, and physical activity. It's also a step toward taking greater responsibility for their health and the health of their future family.

In summary, caring for sperm quality is not just about fertility—it's a fundamental aspect of self-care. Healthy sperm are a reflection of a healthy body and mind, and improving their quality often leads to better quality of life in many areas. It's an investment that pays off both in the short and long term—from higher chances of fatherhood to better health and daily well-being.

Modern challenges in male reproductive health

Male reproductive health, though vital to both societal and biological functions, is increasingly facing challenges stemming from a rapidly changing world. Lifestyle factors, technological advancements, environmental pollution, and societal and professional pressures are now some of the leading contributors to declining sperm quality and overall reproductive health. Today's men grapple with issues that were neither as widespread nor as intense a few decades ago.

One of the primary challenges is the pervasive presence of stress. Living in constant motion, balancing career demands, and meeting societal expectations have left men feeling chronically fatigued and tense. Stress significantly impacts reproductive health by elevating cortisol levels—a hormone that suppresses testosterone production. Testosterone, the key male hormone, is essential for a healthy reproductive system, and its deficiency can lead to reduced sperm quality, diminished libido, and other health issues.

Environmental pollution poses another major challenge to reproductive health. Today's men are exposed to toxins like heavy metals, pesticides, and chemicals commonly found in plastics, such as Bisphenol A (BPA). These substances can disrupt hormonal balance, negatively affecting sperm production and quality. Additionally, air pollution, particularly in urban areas, has been shown to decrease sperm motility, further complicating the fertilization process.

Technological advancements and their impact on reproductive health also deserve attention. Modern life is inseparable from electronic devices like smartphones and laptops. These devices emit electromagnetic radiation and heat, which can affect sperm quality. Studies suggest that carrying a phone in your trouser pocket or placing a laptop on your lap can reduce sperm count and motility. While technology simplifies life, improper usage can have unintended health consequences.

The modern male lifestyle is another significant factor. Diets high in processed foods, lack of regular exercise, excessive alcohol consumption, and smoking all contribute to declining sperm quality. Processed foods often lack the essential vitamins and minerals needed for sperm production, while substance use further burdens the body, disrupting hormonal balance and reducing reproductive potential.

Modern challenges also extend to health conditions. Lifestyle diseases like obesity, diabetes, and hypertension increasingly affect younger men, negatively impacting their reproductive capacity. Obesity, associated with hormonal imbalances and chronic inflammation, is a leading risk factor for reduced sperm quality. Additionally, sexually transmitted infections, which remain a significant issue, can cause permanent damage to the reproductive system if not diagnosed and treated promptly.

In conclusion, the challenges facing male reproductive health today are multifaceted and stem from a variety of factors. However, understanding these issues is the first step toward change. Education, the adoption of healthy habits, and a conscious approach to lifestyle can significantly improve the situation. Reproductive health is not only an individual concern but also a cornerstone of building a better future—both personally and socially.

Table of contents

Chapter 6:
Building Healthy Habits for the Future............................101

Conclusion..119

Chapter 1:
Understanding Sperm Quality

The modern world presents numerous challenges to male reproductive health. While issues related to fertility are increasingly discussed, the critical role of sperm quality often remains underexplored. This topic, long overshadowed by other health concerns, is of immense importance—not only for men hoping to become fathers but also for their overall health and well-being.

To understand why sperm quality matters so much, we first need to look at what sperm truly represents. Sperm is not just a medium for fertilization—it's a highly complex biological system containing sperm cells and a variety of substances that support their function. These microscopic cells play a pivotal role in reproduction. Their structure, motility, and resilience in challenging environments determine whether fertilization is even possible.

Unfortunately, global statistics reveal a worrying trend: the quality of sperm among men worldwide is declining. Studies indicate a reduction in sperm count per ejaculate, along with decreases in motility and morphology. What's causing this trend? It turns out that contemporary lifestyles, stress, environmental pollution, and even dietary habits can significantly impact reproductive health. Understanding these factors is the first step toward addressing the problem.

However, discussing sperm quality isn't just about fertility. Sperm quality serves as a mirror reflecting a man's overall health. Many health issues, such as hormonal imbalances, chronic illnesses, or obesity, directly impact the reproductive system. Taking care of sperm quality, therefore, isn't solely about future fatherhood—it's also about prioritizing personal health and longevity.

Chapter 1 of this book is dedicated to thoroughly examining what sperm is and the functions it performs. You'll learn about the sperm lifecycle, the critical parameters of sperm health, and why monitoring them is essential. We'll also discuss common problems men face and how to identify and address them. This knowledge is crucial for understanding your own body and making informed decisions about reproductive health.

Understanding sperm quality lays the groundwork for the steps discussed in subsequent chapters. Without this foundational knowledge, it's difficult to make informed improvements to your health. Our bodies are intricate systems, and each part affects the others. The more we understand about how sperm works, the easier it becomes to implement changes that yield real results.

1.1. What is sperm and why is it important?

Semen, often thought of solely in terms of fertilization, is an intricate and multifaceted biological substance that plays a role far beyond its obvious reproductive function. It is the medium through which sperm is delivered, but its importance stretches into the realms of genetics, overall health, and even the evolutionary success of the human species. Understanding what semen is and why it matters requires a deeper look at its composition, its role in reproduction, and the factors that affect its quality.

At the heart of semen's role are sperm cells, the primary carriers of male genetic material. Each sperm cell is a marvel of biological engineering, designed to perform the critical task of fertilization. Sperm are composed of three key parts: the head, which houses the DNA; the midpiece, which contains mitochondria to fuel movement; and the tail, or flagellum, which propels the sperm toward the egg. The ability of sperm to move efficiently, known as motility, is a key factor in successful fertilization. However, beyond motility, other qualities like morphology (shape) and viability (ability to survive) play critical roles. A healthy sperm must have an intact head, a properly functioning midpiece, and a strong tail to navigate the journey to the egg.

While sperm is a vital component of semen, it is only one part of a more complex system. Seminal fluid, produced by various glands including the prostate and seminal vesicles, acts as a carrier and protector for sperm. This fluid is rich in enzymes, proteins, sugars such as fructose, and substances that modulate immune responses. These components are essential for nourishing the sperm and providing them with the energy needed to survive in the female reproductive tract, where conditions can be hostile. For instance, the acidic environment of the vagina can be detrimental to sperm, and the alkaline nature of seminal fluid helps neutralize this acidity.

Another crucial role of seminal fluid is its ability to enhance sperm motility and aid in their transport. It acts as a lubricant and medium through which sperm can move efficiently. Additionally, the fluid contains antioxidants that help protect sperm from oxidative stress, a damaging process caused by free radicals. Oxidative stress can lead to DNA fragmentation in sperm, reducing their ability to fertilize an egg or potentially leading to genetic issues in offspring.

The production of semen, including sperm, is a complex biological process known as spermatogenesis. This process occurs in the testes and is regulated by hormones such as testosterone and follicle-stimulating hormone (FSH). Spermatogenesis is a continuous cycle where stem cells develop into mature sperm over approximately 64 days. These newly formed sperm then travel to the epididymis, where they undergo further maturation, gaining the ability to swim and fertilize an egg. However, this process is highly sensitive to external factors such as temperature, hormonal imbalances, and lifestyle habits, which can all affect sperm production and quality.

Semen quality is not only a reflection of reproductive health but also a mirror of overall physical well-being. Poor semen quality can indicate underlying health issues, such as hormonal imbalances, chronic stress, or exposure to environmental toxins. For example, low testosterone levels, often linked to sedentary lifestyles or obesity, can result in reduced sperm production and lower motility. Similarly, exposure to harmful substances like pesticides, heavy metals, or endocrine-disrupting chemicals can negatively impact both the quantity and quality of sperm.

Genetically, semen plays a pivotal role in the creation of new life. Each sperm carries a unique set of genes, which, when combined with the genetic material of the egg, form the blueprint for a new individual. This makes the genetic integrity of sperm critically important. Factors such as oxidative damage, poor diet, smoking, or excessive alcohol consumption can harm sperm DNA, increasing the likelihood of infertility or potential health complications for offspring.

Beyond its biological and genetic significance, semen also holds a place in the broader context of male health and lifestyle. Healthy semen production is influenced by a range of factors, including diet, physical activity, sleep, and stress management. Diets rich in antioxidants, vitamins, and minerals, for instance, can improve sperm quality, while regular exercise helps maintain hormonal balance. Conversely, unhealthy habits such as smoking, excessive drinking, or poor dietary choices can severely impact semen quality and overall reproductive health.

Interestingly, semen is also studied in the context of evolutionary biology. The ability of sperm to compete for fertilization, a phenomenon known as sperm competition, highlights its role in human reproduction. Seminal fluid contains proteins that can influence the female reproductive environment, increasing the chances of successful fertilization. This evolutionary perspective underscores the complexity and importance of semen in the survival of the species.

In summary, semen is far more than just a carrier of sperm—it is a complex, multifunctional biological substance essential for reproduction, genetic integrity, and overall male health. Its quality is influenced by a wide array of factors, from hormonal health and lifestyle habits to environmental conditions and dietary choices. Understanding what semen is and why it matters is not only crucial for those planning to start a family but also for any man looking to take control of his reproductive health and well-being. Taking care of semen quality is an investment in the future, reflecting not just the ability to conceive but the broader aspects of vitality, health, and longevity.

1.2. The structure and functions of sperm

Sperm, despite their microscopic size, are among the most complex and specialized cells in the human body. Their structure and functions have been meticulously designed to fulfill one of the most critical biological roles: fertilizing an egg. Understanding the anatomy of sperm and the mechanisms that drive their functionality provides crucial insights into why sperm quality is so essential for reproductive health.

Each sperm cell consists of three main parts: the head, the midpiece, and the tail. The head is the most important part of the sperm as it contains the genetic material—DNA. This DNA carries the father's genetic information, which merges with the mother's DNA during fertilization to create a unique genetic blueprint for a new individual. The sperm head also contains the acrosome, a structure filled with enzymes that help the sperm penetrate the egg's protective outer layer. The integrity of the sperm head is critical for successful fertilization, as any abnormalities can hinder the sperm's ability to perform its role.

The midpiece of the sperm, often referred to as the "powerhouse," is home to mitochondria. These energy-producing structures provide the necessary fuel for the sperm to move. This energy is crucial, as the sperm must travel a long and challenging journey through the female reproductive system, navigating the cervix, uterus, and fallopian tubes to reach the egg. The mitochondria in the midpiece serve as the driving force, enabling the sperm to sustain this arduous trek.

The tail, or flagellum, of the sperm is responsible for its movement. Through its whip-like motion, the tail propels the sperm forward in the seminal fluid and through the female reproductive tract. Sperm motility, or the ability to move actively and effectively, is a key factor in fertilization success. Insufficient motility can significantly impede the sperm's chances of reaching the egg, even if their count and morphology are normal.

An essential aspect of sperm functionality is their ability to survive in the challenging environment of the female reproductive system. Sperm must overcome numerous obstacles, including the acidic pH of the vagina and the immune responses of the female body. While seminal fluid provides a protective buffer, the sperm themselves are equipped with adaptive mechanisms that increase their chances of survival and successful fertilization.

Understanding the structure and functions of sperm also highlights the importance of their quality. Factors such as oxidative stress, poor diet, lack of physical activity, or exposure to toxins can damage sperm, affecting their motility, fertilization capability, and DNA integrity. This is why adopting a healthy lifestyle and avoiding harmful influences are vital for improving reproductive health.

In summary, sperm are a testament to biological precision. Their structure and functions are intricately linked to their ability to fulfill their ultimate purpose: passing on life. Recognizing these mechanisms is the first step toward consciously caring for sperm quality and overall reproductive health.

1.3. Key sperm parameters: count, motility, morphology

The quality of semen, while largely influenced by a man's overall health, is primarily assessed through three key parameters: quantity, motility, and morphology of sperm. These indicators directly impact a sperm's ability to fertilize an egg, and their analysis forms the cornerstone of male fertility diagnostics. Each of these parameters plays a vital role in the reproductive process, and understanding them sheds light on why maintaining healthy semen is so crucial.

The first and most basic parameter is **sperm quantity**—the number of sperm present in semen. According to the World Health Organization (WHO), a sperm concentration of at least 15 million sperm per milliliter of semen is considered normal. However, quantity alone does not guarantee fertility. Even if the sperm count is high, their quality, including motility and morphology, must also meet certain standards. A condition known as oligospermia refers to low sperm count, which significantly reduces the likelihood of fertilization. In more severe cases, azoospermia, the complete absence of sperm in semen, makes natural conception impossible.

The second crucial factor is **sperm motility**, or their ability to actively move toward the egg. Motility is what enables sperm to navigate the challenging journey through the female reproductive tract, including the cervix, uterus, and fallopian tubes. Sperm motility is classified into different categories, ranging from progressive motility—where sperm move effectively in a straight line—to non-progressive or aimless motion, which is not conducive to fertilization. WHO guidelines suggest that at least 32% of sperm in a sample should exhibit progressive motility to be considered healthy. Reduced motility, known as asthenozoospermia, significantly decreases the chances of natural fertilization.

The third parameter is **sperm morphology**, or the shape and structure of the sperm. A healthy sperm should have an oval head, a proportional midpiece, and a straight, flexible tail. Any deviations from this norm, such as an abnormally large head, irregularly shaped midpiece, or damaged tail, can impair a sperm's ability to fertilize an egg. Studies show that even minor abnormalities in sperm morphology can impact their motility and ability to penetrate the egg's protective layers. According to WHO standards, semen is considered normal if at least 4% of sperm have an ideal structure.

These three parameters—quantity, motility, and morphology—are closely interrelated. For instance, even if the sperm count is high, low motility or abnormal morphology can significantly reduce the chances of successful fertilization. This is why a comprehensive evaluation of semen quality is essential in diagnosing male fertility. The results of such analyses can provide insights into potential health issues, such as hormonal imbalances, inflammation, or the adverse effects of environmental factors.

Semen quality is also dynamic and can change in response to lifestyle, diet, or exposure to toxins. Healthy habits, such as a balanced diet rich in antioxidants, regular exercise, and avoiding harmful substances, can significantly improve all three parameters. Conversely, stress, sleep deprivation, poor diet, and exposure to harmful chemicals can lower semen quality, affecting sperm quantity, motility, and morphology.

In conclusion, the quantity, motility, and morphology of sperm are critical indicators of male reproductive health. Understanding and taking steps to improve these parameters can not only increase the chances of conception but also enhance a man's overall health and well-being.

1.4. The sperm life cycle: from production to maturity

The life cycle of sperm, from its genesis in the testes to reaching full maturity, is one of the most precise and intricate processes in the human body. Known as spermatogenesis, this process involves multiple stages during which stem cells transform into mature sperm capable of fertilizing an egg. Understanding this cycle underscores the importance of maintaining optimal environmental and health conditions for male reproductive well-being.

Sperm production begins in the testes, specifically within tiny structures called seminiferous tubules. These microscopic tubes serve as the site where stem cells, known as spermatogonia, begin their transformation. Under the influence of hormones like testosterone and follicle-stimulating hormone (FSH), spermatogonia divide and undergo a series of changes, eventually becoming spermatocytes and then spermatids. This phase, called spermatogenesis, takes approximately 64 days, though individual variations may occur based on health and environmental factors.

A pivotal moment in spermatogenesis is the process of cellular division, during which the chromosome count is halved to 23. This reduction ensures that each sperm carries a unique genetic code, ready to merge with the egg's DNA and create a genetically diverse offspring. It is at this stage that abnormalities, such as genetic mutations or errors in cellular division, can occur, potentially affecting sperm quality and reproductive success.

Once spermatogenesis is complete, sperm are not yet fully functional. They move to the epididymis, a structure adjacent to the testes, where they undergo a crucial maturation phase. The epididymis serves as a "training ground" for sperm, where they gain the ability to move by developing a functioning tail and finalize their morphological structure. During this weeks-long process, sperm also adapt to surviving in seminal fluid and prepare for the challenges of navigating the female reproductive tract.

Mature sperm are stored in the epididymis, where they remain viable for several days until ejaculation. During ejaculation, sperm are mixed with secretions from the prostate and seminal vesicles, forming semen. This fluid plays a protective and nutritive role, enabling sperm to survive the hostile environment of the female reproductive system. Interestingly, if sperm are not utilized for fertilization, the body naturally reabsorbs them and replaces them with newly produced cells.

The sperm life cycle is highly sensitive to external factors. Stress, unhealthy diets, physical inactivity, and exposure to toxins can all negatively affect the quantity and quality of sperm produced. High temperatures, such as those caused by overheating the testes, can also disrupt spermatogenesis, making it essential to avoid prolonged use of tight clothing or frequent hot baths.

It is important to note that sperm production is a lifelong process, although sperm quality and quantity may decline with age. Regular health check-ups, maintaining a healthy lifestyle, and avoiding harmful habits are essential for preserving high-quality semen and reproductive health.

In summary, the life cycle of sperm is a fascinating biological process that plays a crucial role in reproduction. Each stage—from production in the testes, maturation in the epididymis, to ejaculation—requires optimal health and environmental conditions. Understanding these mechanisms empowers men to take better care of their reproductive health and make informed decisions in their daily lives.

1.5. Factors that influence sperm quality

Sperm quality is influenced by a multitude of factors that can either enhance or impair male reproductive health. Semen is particularly sensitive to environmental changes, lifestyle habits, diet, and overall health. Each of these elements directly impacts parameters such as sperm count, motility, and morphology.

Diet plays a pivotal role in sperm quality. Like every other cell in the body, sperm requires the right nutrients to function properly. Antioxidants such as vitamin C, vitamin E, and beta-carotene are essential for protecting sperm from oxidative stress, which can damage their DNA. Minerals like zinc and selenium are crucial for sperm production and improving motility. Conversely, diets rich in saturated fats, simple sugars, and processed foods can lower sperm quality. A lack of essential vitamins and minerals may lead to reduced sperm count and fertility potential.

Lifestyle choices are another significant factor. Smoking, excessive alcohol consumption, and drug use negatively affect sperm production. Nicotine and chemicals in cigarette smoke can damage sperm DNA and reduce motility. Alcohol, especially in large quantities, disrupts hormonal balance, leading to decreased sperm production. Drugs such as marijuana and cocaine not only lower sperm count but also contribute to abnormal morphology.

Stress and lack of sleep have a profound impact on sperm quality. Elevated cortisol levels, the body's primary stress hormone, can suppress testosterone production, which is essential for spermatogenesis. Inadequate sleep affects the body's ability to recover and maintain hormonal balance, further reducing sperm quality. Chronic stress and fatigue can decrease energy levels and increase oxidative stress, which may damage sperm cells.

Environmental factors play an increasingly significant role in male reproductive health. Air pollution, exposure to pesticides, and chemicals found in plastics (e.g., bisphenol A) can disrupt hormonal balance and reduce sperm quality. Prolonged heat exposure, such as frequent sauna use, hot baths, or wearing tight clothing, can also negatively impact sperm production. Elevated testicular temperature interferes with spermatogenesis, lowering sperm count and motility.

Physical activity has both positive and negative effects. Regular moderate exercise can improve sperm quality by promoting hormonal balance, reducing stress, and enhancing blood circulation. However, excessive training, especially to the point of overtraining, may lower testosterone levels and negatively affect sperm production. Additionally, the use of anabolic steroids by athletes or bodybuilders can cause permanent damage to the reproductive system.

Health conditions such as obesity, diabetes, and infections of the genitourinary system also significantly affect sperm quality. Obesity is associated with hormonal imbalances that reduce sperm production. Diabetes, particularly when poorly managed, can damage blood vessels and nerves, impairing testicular function. Infections like orchitis or prostatitis can reduce sperm count and motility.

Each of these factors affects sperm in unique ways, but they often act synergistically—one negative element can amplify the effects of another. This highlights the importance of maintaining a healthy lifestyle, avoiding harmful habits, and minimizing exposure to environmental risks.

1.6. Common sperm issues: from low count to reduced motility

Semen quality issues affect an increasing number of men globally, and their causes are often multifaceted. The most common problems include low sperm count, reduced motility, and abnormal morphology. Each of these issues significantly impacts fertility and serves as a critical indicator of male reproductive health.

One of the most prevalent issues is **low sperm count**, medically referred to as oligospermia. According to the World Health Organization (WHO), a sperm concentration of at least 15 million sperm per milliliter of semen is considered normal. In cases of oligospermia, this number is significantly lower, which reduces the likelihood of successful fertilization. The causes of low sperm count are varied, ranging from hormonal imbalances, such as low testosterone levels, to environmental factors, such as exposure to toxins. Stress, poor diet, and physical inactivity are also major contributors to decreased sperm production.

Another critical issue is **reduced sperm motility**, known as asthenozoospermia. Motility is crucial for sperm to travel through the cervix, uterus, and fallopian tubes to reach the egg. Low motility means that sperm move slowly or in an uncoordinated manner, significantly hindering fertilization. Causes of asthenozoospermia include oxidative stress, infections of the reproductive tract, and exposure to high temperatures that disrupt the normal process of spermatogenesis. For instance, frequent use of saunas or tight clothing can elevate testicular temperatures, negatively impacting sperm function.

Abnormal sperm morphology, or shape, is another factor affecting semen quality. A healthy sperm should have an oval head, a proportional midpiece, and a straight, flexible tail. Deviations from this norm, such as double-headed sperm, improperly shaped tails, or defects in the head, can impair the sperm's ability to penetrate the egg. Factors influencing morphology include genetic disorders, oxidative stress, and exposure to environmental toxins such as pesticides and heavy metals.

Infections in the reproductive system, such as prostatitis, epididymitis, or bacterial infections, play a significant role in semen quality issues. These infections can cause inflammation that damages sperm and disrupts their maturation process. In many cases, such infections remain undetected for extended periods, exacerbating fertility problems. For example, untreated infections can lead to scarring or blockages in the sperm ducts, further complicating natural conception.

Hormonal imbalances, including low testosterone levels or dysfunctions in the pituitary gland, are also major contributors to poor semen quality. Testosterone is a critical hormone responsible for spermatogenesis, and its deficiency can lead to reduced sperm production and motility. Hormonal imbalances may result from medical conditions such as hypogonadism or be side effects of certain medications or anabolic steroid use. Long-term use of steroids, for instance, can suppress the body's natural hormone production, leading to infertility.

Lifestyle factors significantly influence semen quality as well. Smoking, excessive alcohol consumption, lack of physical activity, and an unhealthy diet all contribute to declining sperm health. Cigarette smoking introduces harmful chemicals that damage sperm DNA, while excessive alcohol consumption disrupts hormonal balance and impairs the body's natural repair mechanisms. Diets lacking essential nutrients, such as zinc, selenium, and antioxidants, further exacerbate these issues, reducing sperm count, motility, and morphology.

Finally, psychological factors such as chronic stress and sleep deprivation can negatively impact semen quality. Elevated cortisol levels, the body's primary stress hormone, suppress testosterone production and disrupt the hormonal environment necessary for healthy sperm production. Sleep deprivation compounds this issue by reducing the body's ability to repair cellular damage, including that affecting sperm cells.

By understanding the multifaceted nature of these issues, men can take proactive steps to improve their reproductive health. From making lifestyle changes to seeking medical advice, addressing the underlying causes of semen quality problems is essential for improving fertility and overall well-being.

Chapter 2:
Lifestyle and Reproductive Health

Lifestyle is the foundation of our health—it affects our well-being, energy levels, resilience to stress, and, importantly, reproductive health. When it comes to sperm quality, lifestyle choices play a particularly crucial role, as daily habits can either support the production of healthy sperm or hinder it. Eating habits, physical activity levels, stress management skills, and approaches to substances like alcohol or tobacco are all factors that determine how well the reproductive system functions.

Today's world presents men with many challenges. Long work hours, lack of time for rest, stressful situations, and easy access to unhealthy food are just a few of the problems we face. Each of these factors can have a potentially negative impact on reproductive health, lowering sperm quality and reducing the chances of fatherhood. Fortunately, lifestyle is an area where we have full control—even small changes can yield significant results.

One of the most critical lifestyle factors affecting sperm health is diet. What we eat provides the body with essential nutrients that support sperm production and function. Deficiencies in vitamins and minerals can lead to decreased sperm quality, while a diet rich in antioxidants and healthy fats enhances motility and fertility. A man's diet when planning fatherhood should be thoughtful yet practical and easy to implement on a daily basis.

Equally important is physical activity. Regular exercise helps maintain a healthy weight, improves blood circulation, and supports hormonal balance, which is crucial for reproductive health. However, excessive physical exertion, especially when combined with poor nutrition, can have the opposite effect. Finding a balance between activity and recovery is key to achieving optimal results.

Stress is another factor that significantly impacts sperm quality. High stress levels increase the production of cortisol, a hormone that negatively affects testosterone production and sperm health. Additionally, stress often leads to unhealthy coping mechanisms such as smoking or alcohol consumption, which further burden the body. Learning how to manage psychological tension is one of the most important skills for supporting reproductive health.

Chapter 2 of this book will explore how lifestyle can either support or weaken a man's health. You'll learn which foods to include in your diet, which exercises are most beneficial, and how to manage stress while reducing the impact of harmful substances on the body. We'll also discuss how sleep and recovery influence sperm production and why regular health check-ups are essential. Lifestyle is a tool that allows you to take control of your own health—all it takes is a bit of willingness to start making positive changes.

2.1. Diet for healthy sperm: what to eat and what to avoid

A healthy diet plays a crucial role in maintaining sperm quality and male reproductive health. Sperm, like every other cell in the body, require proper nutrients to function effectively. A well-balanced diet can enhance sperm motility, increase their count, and protect genetic material from damage. Conversely, poor eating habits can lead to significant reproductive health issues.

One of the most critical dietary components for sperm health is **antioxidants**, which protect cells from oxidative stress. Oxidative stress is a leading cause of DNA damage in sperm and reduced motility. Foods rich in antioxidants, such as berries (strawberries, blueberries, raspberries), leafy greens (spinach, kale), and nuts, should be staples in the diet of any man concerned with his reproductive health. Vitamins C and E, found in citrus fruits, almonds, and avocados, are particularly important as they strengthen sperm cell membranes, shielding them from harmful free radicals.

Omega-3 fatty acids are another essential part of a sperm-friendly diet. These fats support the flexibility of sperm cell membranes and enhance their motility. Omega-3s are abundant in fatty fish like salmon, mackerel, and sardines, as well as in walnuts and flaxseeds. Regular consumption of these foods positively influences spermatogenesis, boosting the production of healthy sperm.

A diet rich in **zinc and selenium** is equally vital for the male reproductive system. Zinc, found in meat, seafood (especially oysters), and pumpkin seeds, supports testosterone production, a hormone crucial for spermatogenesis. Selenium, present in Brazil nuts, eggs, and fish, improves sperm motility and protects them from oxidative damage.

It's also important to limit the intake of **simple sugars and processed foods**, which can cause inflammation in the body and lower sperm quality. Fast foods, sugary snacks, and carbonated drinks not only negatively affect body weight but also disrupt hormonal balance, directly impacting sperm production.

Alcohol and caffeine, when consumed excessively, can also impair sperm quality. While moderate coffee consumption may have some health benefits, too much caffeine can disrupt hormonal balance. Alcohol, especially in large quantities, lowers testosterone levels and can lead to DNA damage in sperm. Therefore, reducing the intake of these substances is essential for supporting reproductive health.

A diet for healthy sperm should include whole grains, legumes, and high-quality proteins such as poultry, fish, or tofu. These provide essential amino acids and energy for metabolic processes in reproductive cells. Staying well-hydrated is also crucial, as proper hydration improves the quality of seminal fluid.

Adopting healthy eating habits can yield noticeable benefits in a relatively short time. Within just a few weeks of following a proper diet, improvements in sperm parameters such as count and motility can become evident. Consistency and avoiding harmful factors are key to maximizing the positive effects of a healthy diet.

2.2. The importance of physical activity for fertility

Physical activity plays a vital role in maintaining overall health and improving sperm quality and male fertility. Regular exercise not only supports the proper functioning of the hormonal system but also helps maintain an optimal weight, reduces stress, and enhances blood circulation. All these factors are directly linked to the process of spermatogenesis and the ability of sperm to perform effectively.

One of the most critical aspects of physical activity in the context of reproductive health is its impact on **testosterone levels**. Testosterone, the primary male sex hormone, is essential for the production of sperm. Research shows that moderate physical activities such as jogging, swimming, or strength training can boost testosterone levels, thereby improving sperm quality. However, overly intense workouts, such as marathons or prolonged high-intensity training, can have the opposite effect, leading to overtraining and a drop in testosterone levels.

Physical activity also affects **body weight**, which is a significant factor in assessing male reproductive health. Obesity and overweight can negatively impact sperm quality through hormonal imbalances, such as lower testosterone levels and increased estrogen levels in the body. Regular exercise helps reduce excess body fat and supports hormonal balance, improving sperm parameters such as count and motility.

Blood circulation is another health aspect positively influenced by physical activity. Proper blood flow to the testes is essential for spermatogenesis, as it delivers the nutrients and oxygen required for sperm production. Exercises such as cycling or walking can enhance blood flow, but it's important to note that prolonged pressure on the pelvic area (e.g., from excessive cycling) can have a negative impact on reproductive health.

Physical activity also significantly contributes to **stress reduction**, which is one of the primary factors lowering sperm quality. Exercise stimulates the release of endorphins, commonly known as "feel-good hormones," which help lower cortisol levels—the stress hormone. Reduced stress levels promote better hormonal regulation and improved functioning of the reproductive system.

Choosing the right type and intensity of exercise is crucial for physical activity to benefit reproductive health. Moderate workouts such as brisk walking, yoga, or swimming are ideal, as they do not overly strain the body while supporting overall health. Avoiding extreme physical exertion and ensuring proper recovery is important, as overtraining can increase oxidative stress, which damages sperm.

Appropriate sportswear should not be overlooked. Tight clothing that causes overheating in the testicular area can negatively affect spermatogenesis. Opting for loose, breathable attire, especially during intense workouts, is recommended.

Physical activity is one of the simplest and most natural ways to support male reproductive health. Regular, moderate exercise can significantly improve sperm quality, enhance the chances of conception, and bring benefits to overall well-being and health.

2.3. Stress and sperm quality: managing tension effectively

Stress is one of the most significant factors negatively impacting male reproductive health. In today's world, filled with professional challenges, personal tensions, and societal pressures, stress has become nearly unavoidable. However, excessive and chronic stress can lead to serious consequences, including reduced sperm quality, which can affect fertility.

The mechanism by which stress influences sperm quality begins in the hormonal system. In response to tension, the body releases cortisol, commonly known as the "stress hormone." While cortisol is a natural response to short-term threats, prolonged stress can keep cortisol levels elevated. High cortisol suppresses testosterone production, the primary hormone responsible for spermatogenesis—the process of sperm production. Low testosterone levels can result in decreased sperm count, reduced motility, and a higher risk of DNA damage.

Stress also acts at the cellular level, increasing oxidative stress. This condition arises from an excess of free radicals in the body, which can damage cells, including sperm. Oxidative stress is one of the leading causes of reduced sperm motility and quality and can lead to DNA fragmentation, lowering the chances of conceiving a healthy child.

Chronic stress also affects lifestyle habits, further worsening sperm quality. Stressed individuals often resort to unhealthy coping mechanisms such as smoking, excessive alcohol consumption, poor diet, or physical inactivity. These behaviors are harmful to reproductive health on their own, and combined with stress, they can exacerbate the damage.

Managing stress is a critical component of improving sperm quality and overall reproductive health. Several effective methods can help reduce tension. One of these is meditation, which calms the mind and lowers cortisol levels. Regular meditation practice can improve hormonal balance and reduce stress's negative impact on spermatogenesis.

Deep breathing techniques are another effective method for stress reduction. By activating the parasympathetic nervous system responsible for relaxation, even a few minutes of mindful breathing daily can yield noticeable benefits in lowering stress levels. Progressive muscle relaxation, which involves systematically tensing and relaxing muscle groups, also helps calm the body.

Physical activity is another powerful way to combat stress. Regular exercise, such as running, yoga, or walking in nature, stimulates the release of endorphins, often called "feel-good hormones." Endorphins help lower cortisol levels and improve overall well-being, indirectly benefiting sperm quality.

Emotional support from loved ones also plays a vital role in coping with stress. Conversations with a partner, friends, or a therapist can help alleviate emotional tension and provide new perspectives on challenging situations. It's essential not to ignore emotions and seek support when needed.

Incorporating healthy habits into daily life, such as maintaining regular sleep, eating a balanced diet, and limiting stimulants, also reduces the impact of stress on the body. Avoiding caffeine and alcohol before bedtime can improve sleep quality, which in turn supports the recovery of the reproductive system.

Reducing stress is not an easy task, but its effects can be seen not only in improved sperm quality but also in overall well-being and mental health. Taking conscious steps toward managing tension can bring significant benefits in both the short and long term.

2.4. Alcohol, smoking, and other substances and their impact on fertility

Lifestyle choices have a profound impact on male reproductive health, and one of the most critical factors is avoiding substances such as alcohol, tobacco, and other psychoactive drugs. These habits, while seemingly harmless in the short term, have long-term and detrimental effects on sperm quality and the ability to conceive. The impact of these substances on the male reproductive system is multifaceted, affecting both sperm parameters and overall hormonal balance.

Alcohol is one of the most widely consumed psychoactive substances globally, but its impact on sperm quality is significantly negative, especially when consumed in excess. Regular alcohol consumption lowers testosterone levels, the hormone crucial for sperm production. Additionally, alcohol disrupts the body's hormonal balance, leading to reduced sperm count, lower motility, and an increase in abnormal sperm morphology. Furthermore, alcohol metabolites, such as acetaldehyde, can cause DNA damage in sperm, thereby reducing their fertilization potential.

Cigarettes, which contain thousands of harmful chemicals including nicotine and heavy metals, are equally destructive to male reproductive health. Smoking causes oxidative stress in the body, a major contributor to sperm damage. Oxidative stress leads to decreased sperm motility and DNA fragmentation. Studies show that men who smoke have significantly reduced sperm parameters compared to nonsmokers, which can substantially lower their chances of natural conception.

Other psychoactive substances, such as marijuana, cocaine, and amphetamines, also negatively affect sperm quality. Marijuana, often perceived as less harmful, disrupts testosterone production and reduces sperm count and motility. Cocaine and amphetamines, which stimulate the nervous system, can cause severe damage to the blood vessels in the testes, reducing the body's ability to produce healthy sperm. Prolonged use of these substances can result in permanent damage to the reproductive system.

The effects of these substances on fertility extend beyond sperm parameters. Regular use of alcohol, cigarettes, or drugs can lead to overall health decline, including erectile dysfunction, libido problems, and reduced physical endurance. These substances also impact the health of future offspring—DNA damage in sperm increases the risk of genetic abnormalities in children.

It is important to emphasize that the effects of these substances on reproductive health are largely reversible if appropriate lifestyle changes are made. Quitting smoking, reducing alcohol consumption, and avoiding other psychoactive substances can significantly improve sperm quality within a few months. The reproductive system regenerates relatively quickly, and sperm produced after substance cessation are typically much healthier.

Awareness of the negative impact of substances on fertility and taking steps to reduce or eliminate their use is crucial for improving reproductive health. A healthy lifestyle, including a balanced diet, physical activity, and abstaining from harmful habits, can greatly increase the chances of conception and improve overall well-being.

2.5. Sleep and recovery: why rest is crucial

Sleep is a fundamental element of a healthy lifestyle and is vital for overall well-being, bodily functions, and male reproductive health. The fast-paced modern lifestyle, filled with responsibilities and tensions, often leads to neglecting the quantity and quality of sleep. Unfortunately, chronic sleep deprivation has serious consequences, including reduced sperm quality, decreased testosterone levels, and impaired regenerative processes essential for reproductive system functioning.

During sleep, the body cycles through various stages that play a crucial role in physical and mental recovery. One of the most important stages is deep sleep, also known as slow-wave sleep. It is during this phase that testosterone—a hormone essential for spermatogenesis—is produced. Regular sleep helps maintain adequate testosterone levels, positively influencing sperm count, motility, and genetic quality. Interrupting the sleep cycle or lacking sufficient rest can lead to decreased testosterone levels, directly impacting sperm parameters.

Inadequate sleep also impairs the body's ability to reduce oxidative stress, a major factor in sperm damage. During sleep, the body produces melatonin, a hormone that not only regulates the sleep-wake cycle but also acts as a powerful antioxidant. Melatonin helps neutralize free radicals, which can damage sperm DNA, reduce motility, and worsen morphology. Individuals suffering from chronic sleep deprivation often exhibit elevated oxidative stress levels, negatively affecting reproductive health.

A lack of sufficient rest also disrupts hormonal balance. In addition to lowering testosterone levels, chronic sleep deprivation can increase cortisol, the stress hormone. High cortisol levels not only inhibit testosterone production but also interfere with regenerative processes in the testes, making it harder for the body to produce healthy sperm. Furthermore, excess cortisol can negatively impact libido and the ability to maintain erections, compounding fertility issues.

Nightly rest is also essential for the cardiovascular system, which plays a key role in delivering nutrients and oxygen to the testes. During sleep, the circulatory system undergoes repair, allowing for more efficient blood flow to organs. Chronic sleep deprivation can lead to cardiovascular problems, which in turn can disrupt spermatogenesis.

Sleep hygiene, a set of practices that support healthy and restorative sleep, is a critical component of reproductive health. To improve sleep quality, it is important to maintain a consistent schedule —going to bed and waking up at the same time every day, including weekends. Avoiding screens that emit blue light at least an hour before sleep is also important, as blue light suppresses melatonin production. The bedroom should be well-prepared—dark, quiet, and at an optimal temperature. A comfortable bed and breathable bedding are equally important.

Physical activity during the day supports healthy sleep, but intense workouts just before bed should be avoided as they can elevate adrenaline levels, making it harder to fall asleep. Diet also plays a role —avoiding caffeine and heavy meals before bedtime can improve the quality of nightly rest.

An adequate amount of sleep, typically ranging from 7 to 9 hours per night, is essential for reproductive health and overall well-being. Sleep is not just a time for physical recovery but also for restoring the body's reproductive capacity. Adopting healthy sleep habits can significantly improve sperm quality, boost energy levels, and positively impact intimate relationships.

2.6. The role of regular health check-ups and monitoring

Regular health check-ups and monitoring play a crucial role in maintaining sperm quality and overall male reproductive health. While many men tend to avoid visiting the doctor, systematic health assessments can help detect issues early and enable the implementation of preventive or therapeutic measures. Reproductive health is not an isolated aspect—it is closely linked to the overall condition of the body, and regular check-ups provide valuable insights into general well-being.

One of the most important tests for men planning to have children is a **semen analysis**, also known as a spermogram. This test evaluates key sperm parameters, such as count, motility, and morphology. Regular semen analysis is especially important for couples experiencing difficulty conceiving. It provides precise data that can identify potential issues and guide interventions to improve fertility.

Hormonal testing is another essential aspect of monitoring reproductive health. Testosterone, the key hormone for spermatogenesis, must be maintained at an appropriate level. Hormonal imbalances, such as low testosterone or elevated estrogen levels, can significantly reduce sperm quality. Regular blood tests can detect these changes, allowing for lifestyle modifications, supplementation, or hormonal treatments to address the issue.

The health of the **genitourinary system** directly affects sperm quality. Infections such as epididymitis, prostatitis, or urinary tract infections can decrease sperm count and motility. Regular visits to a urologist help detect these issues early, increasing the likelihood of effective treatment and preventing long-term complications.

Obesity and overweight are additional factors that can negatively impact reproductive health. Regular assessments, such as measuring body mass index (BMI) and analyzing blood glucose and lipid levels, help evaluate risks associated with excess weight. Excess body fat can lead to hormonal imbalances that affect sperm production. If such problems are identified, doctors can recommend dietary plans, exercise routines, and other lifestyle changes.

Monitoring reproductive health also provides an opportunity to assess the impact of **environmental factors** on the body. Tests can detect the presence of heavy metals or other toxins that negatively affect sperm quality. Identifying these factors allows individuals to take steps to eliminate them from their daily lives.

Regular health check-ups are also vital for preventive care. Early detection of health issues such as diabetes, hypertension, or cardiovascular diseases enables timely intervention, reducing the risk of further complications. The overall health of the body directly influences the functioning of the reproductive system, making comprehensive health assessments essential.

It is equally important to discuss reproductive health openly with a healthcare provider. Many issues related to sperm quality can have genetic, hormonal, or environmental origins, and a specialist can help understand these connections and suggest personalized solutions.

Systematic health monitoring and regular check-ups are not only key to maintaining sperm quality but also to improving overall well-being and quality of life. A responsible approach to reproductive health is an investment in the future—both personal and for future generations.

Chapter 3:
Environmental Factors

We live in an era where the impact of the environment on our health is increasingly evident. The air we breathe, the chemicals in the products around us, and even the electronic devices we use daily can significantly affect our bodies. Male reproductive health is no exception —environmental factors play a key role in determining sperm quality and the ability of sperm to function properly.

Modern scientific research has shown that the quality of the air we breathe directly affects sperm production and quality. Pollutants such as particulate matter, heavy metals, and chemical compounds found in exhaust fumes can enter the body, disrupting hormonal balance and burdening the reproductive system. Men living in large cities, where smog is a daily concern, may be particularly vulnerable to the adverse effects of pollution.

Another significant factor is the presence of chemicals in everyday products like cosmetics, cleaning supplies, and plastic packaging. Many of these contain endocrine-disrupting substances that can mimic or block the action of natural hormones in the body. Bisphenol A (BPA), phthalates, and pesticides are just a few of the chemicals linked to reduced sperm quality. Awareness of their presence and avoiding them whenever possible are important steps in maintaining reproductive health.

Electronic devices such as smartphones and laptops can also impact sperm quality. This is due to the emission of electromagnetic radiation and heat, which can lower sperm production and motility. It's especially important to limit carrying devices like mobile phones in trouser pockets and to avoid using laptops on your lap for extended periods.

We must also remember the effect of temperature on sperm production. The testes, which are responsible for producing sperm, need to be kept at a lower temperature than the rest of the body. Frequent use of hot baths, saunas, or even wearing tight clothing can lead to overheating, negatively affecting sperm quality.

Chapter 3 of this book focuses on identifying environmental factors that may affect male reproductive health. We'll provide practical tips on minimizing exposure to harmful substances, protecting the body from pollution, and making conscious choices about products and habits that support health. The environment we live in has a significant impact on our bodies, but with the right actions, we can mitigate its negative effects and support reproductive health at every stage of life.

3.1. Air pollution and its impact on sperm

Air pollution is one of the most pressing issues in today's world, and its impact on human health is increasingly well-documented. While much of the focus is on its effects on respiratory and cardiovascular systems, pollution also has a significant influence on male reproductive health. Specifically, prolonged exposure to harmful substances in polluted air can impair sperm quality, reducing fertility potential.

Air pollution consists of fine particulate matter (PM2.5 and PM10), heavy metals, nitrogen oxides, sulfur oxides, and polycyclic aromatic hydrocarbons (PAHs). These harmful substances enter the body through the respiratory system and then circulate in the bloodstream, causing systemic inflammation. This inflammation negatively affects the hormonal system, including testosterone production, which is critical for spermatogenesis. Studies have shown that men living in areas with high air pollution levels are more likely to experience reduced sperm quality, characterized by lower sperm counts, reduced motility, and increased DNA damage.

One of the key mechanisms through which air pollution affects reproductive health is **oxidative stress**. Fine particulate matter triggers an increase in free radicals within the body, which attack cells, including sperm. Damage caused by free radicals includes DNA fragmentation in sperm and abnormalities in their morphology, reducing their fertilization capability. Moreover, oxidative stress can disrupt spermatogenesis processes in the testes, leading to fewer healthy sperm being produced.

Air pollution also disrupts the body's hormonal balance. Exposure to certain chemicals, such as dioxins or PAHs, can act as endocrine disruptors, interfering with hormone production and function. For men, this can result in lower testosterone levels and disturbances in other hormonal processes vital to reproductive health.

Heavy metals like lead, cadmium, and mercury, which are often present in polluted air, also play a role in harming reproductive health. These toxic metals accumulate in the body and can disrupt testicular function and damage sperm at the cellular level. Research shows that even minimal but prolonged exposure to heavy metals can lead to reduced sperm motility and an increase in abnormalities.

Men living in urban areas or near industrial facilities are particularly vulnerable to the harmful effects of air pollution. In such environments, daily exposure to toxic substances can lead to chronic issues with sperm quality. It is essential to take measures to minimize this risk, such as wearing protective masks in highly polluted areas, installing air purifiers at home, and avoiding outdoor activities on days with high smog levels.

Despite the unavoidable exposure to pollution, there are ways to protect reproductive health. A balanced diet rich in antioxidants, such as vitamin C, vitamin E, and selenium, can help neutralize free radicals and reduce oxidative stress. Regular physical activity and a healthy lifestyle also enhance the body's ability to cope with the negative effects of pollution.

Raising awareness about the impact of air pollution on sperm quality and taking protective measures can significantly improve male reproductive health. By paying attention to the quality of the air we breathe, we not only protect our lungs and heart but also secure the future of our families.

3.2. Radiation and electronic devices: facts and myths

In an era of rapid technological advancement and widespread use of electronic devices such as smartphones, laptops, and Wi-Fi routers, concerns about their impact on health—including sperm quality—are increasingly common. The potential harm from electromagnetic radiation emitted by these devices has been the subject of numerous studies, yet myths and uncertainties persist. Understanding the actual risks associated with radiation and how to minimize them is essential.

Electromagnetic radiation (EMF) emitted by electronic devices is a form of energy that travels in waves. Most devices we use daily emit low levels of radiation that are considered safe according to international standards. However, prolonged and close exposure to radiation, particularly near the testes, raises some concerns.

Studies have shown that prolonged use of laptops on one's lap can lead to overheating of the scrotal area. Elevated temperatures in this region directly impact spermatogenesis, the process of sperm production. Sperm are particularly sensitive to heat, requiring a temperature lower than core body temperature to develop properly. Regular exposure to increased heat from laptops may reduce sperm count and impair motility.

Mobile devices such as smartphones also spark controversy regarding reproductive health. Mobile phones emit radio waves, a form of electromagnetic radiation. While the levels are low, keeping a phone in a pants pocket near the reproductive organs for extended periods can increase the temperature in that area and potentially alter sperm quality. While research in this field is still in its early stages, preliminary findings suggest it is prudent to limit the time phones are kept near the testes.

Wi-Fi routers and other wireless devices also emit electromagnetic radiation, but their impact on sperm quality is less clear. Laboratory studies have indicated that prolonged exposure to high levels of Wi-Fi radiation can cause DNA damage in sperm and reduce motility. However, the levels of radiation encountered in daily life are significantly lower than those used in these studies, suggesting that the risk is minimal.

There are also many myths surrounding electromagnetic radiation. One of the most common is the belief that keeping a phone in a pocket always results in irreversible sperm damage. In reality, the impact depends on various factors, including the duration of exposure, the device's proximity to the body, and overall lifestyle. Another myth suggests that using electronic devices at night entirely disrupts the body's regenerative processes. While blue light from screens can affect melatonin production and sleep, there is no direct evidence that electromagnetic radiation alone significantly impacts sperm quality.

To minimize potential risks associated with radiation and electronic devices, several simple practices can be adopted. First, avoid placing laptops directly on your lap—using a stand or placing the device on a desk is an effective way to reduce exposure. Second, try to keep your mobile phone in a bag or jacket pocket rather than pants pockets, especially during prolonged use. Third, if possible, turn off wireless devices at night to minimize exposure during sleep.

In conclusion, while electromagnetic radiation from electronic devices is not a direct cause of severe reproductive issues, responsible use of technology and minimizing exposure can help protect reproductive health. Awareness and good habits can significantly improve sperm quality and overall well-being.

3.3. Chemicals in everyday environments

The modern environment we live in is increasingly filled with chemicals that have the potential to negatively impact human health, including male reproductive health and sperm quality. These compounds, often invisible to the naked eye, are present in the air we breathe, the water we drink, the food we eat, and the products we use every day. While they might seem harmless on the surface, long-term exposure to certain chemicals can lead to significant reproductive health issues. Understanding how these substances affect the body and taking steps to minimize exposure are critical for maintaining sperm quality and overall reproductive health.

One of the most concerning groups of chemicals are **endocrine disruptors**. These substances interfere with the normal functioning of the hormonal system, affecting hormone production, release, and action within the body. Common endocrine disruptors include bisphenol A (BPA) and phthalates, which are found in many everyday items such as plastic containers, food packaging, personal care products, and even children's toys. BPA, in particular, is known to mimic estrogen, a hormone that can disrupt the delicate hormonal balance in men. Exposure to BPA has been linked to reduced testosterone levels, a hormone essential for the production of sperm. Phthalates, on the other hand, can impair spermatogenesis—the process by which sperm are produced—leading to lower sperm counts and motility.

Pesticides and herbicides used in agriculture are another major concern. These chemicals are designed to protect crops from pests and weeds, but their residues often remain on the food we eat and can contaminate drinking water supplies. When consumed over time, these compounds can accumulate in the body, causing toxic effects. Studies have shown that exposure to certain pesticides, such as organophosphates and carbamates, can lead to DNA damage in sperm and disrupt the function of the male reproductive system. This damage not only affects the ability of sperm to fertilize an egg but also increases the risk of transmitting genetic abnormalities to offspring. Opting for organic produce and thoroughly washing fruits and vegetables can help reduce exposure to these harmful substances.

Another significant group of harmful substances includes **heavy metals** such as lead, mercury, and cadmium. These metals are often found in polluted air, water, and soil, and their presence is linked to industrial emissions, old plumbing systems, and even certain types of seafood. Heavy metals have the ability to accumulate in the body over time, causing damage to various organs, including the testes. Lead, for example, has been shown to interfere with sperm production, leading to lower sperm counts and impaired motility. Mercury, commonly found in certain fish like tuna and swordfish, can cause oxidative stress in sperm, leading to DNA fragmentation and other structural damage. Cadmium, often present in cigarette smoke and industrial waste, has similar detrimental effects on male reproductive health. Reducing exposure to heavy metals by avoiding polluted areas, using filtered water, and being mindful of seafood consumption can help protect sperm quality.

Personal care products and cosmetics are another hidden source of harmful chemicals. Many of these products contain parabens and triclosan, which act as preservatives and antimicrobial agents. While these compounds might help extend the shelf life of products, they can also act as endocrine disruptors, interfering with the hormonal balance necessary for sperm production. Choosing natural or organic personal care products can help minimize this risk. Similarly, some cleaning products, air fresheners, and scented candles release volatile organic compounds (VOCs), which can exacerbate oxidative stress in the body and negatively impact sperm health.

Chemicals in household items, such as paints, adhesives, and furniture, can also pose risks. Many of these products release VOCs into the air, especially when new. These compounds can irritate the respiratory system and contribute to systemic oxidative stress, a condition that has been directly linked to decreased sperm quality. Ensuring proper ventilation when using such products and opting for low-VOC or non-toxic alternatives can help mitigate exposure.

The role of oxidative stress in sperm damage cannot be overstated. Many chemicals, whether from pesticides, heavy metals, or VOCs, contribute to the production of free radicals in the body. These unstable molecules attack cellular structures, including the DNA within sperm. Over time, this damage accumulates, reducing sperm motility, count, and the ability to fertilize an egg. Consuming a diet rich in antioxidants —found in foods like berries, nuts, and leafy greens—can help counteract oxidative stress and protect sperm from damage.

Beyond individual choices, understanding the broader sources of chemical exposure is also important. Industrial pollution, for instance, is a significant contributor to the presence of harmful substances in the environment. Men working in industries such as manufacturing, agriculture, or chemical processing are often at a higher risk of exposure to reproductive toxins. Regular health check-ups and occupational safety measures, such as using protective equipment and limiting direct contact with harmful substances, are essential for those in high-risk professions.

Plastic usage is another area where small changes can make a big difference. Many plastic products, especially when heated, can release harmful chemicals like BPA and phthalates. Avoiding microwaving food in plastic containers, using glass or stainless-steel alternatives, and drinking from BPA-free bottles are simple steps that can significantly reduce exposure.

Finally, awareness and education play a vital role in protecting reproductive health from chemical exposure. By staying informed about the potential risks associated with everyday products and making conscious choices to minimize exposure, men can take proactive steps to safeguard their fertility. Simple actions, such as opting for organic foods, using air purifiers, and selecting natural household and personal care products, can collectively have a significant impact on sperm quality and overall reproductive health.

In conclusion, while the modern environment presents numerous challenges to reproductive health due to chemical exposure, there are practical steps that men can take to protect themselves. Awareness, combined with informed lifestyle choices, can help mitigate the effects of these harmful substances, improving sperm quality and supporting long-term reproductive wellness.

3.4. Temperature and sperm production: avoiding overheating

Temperature is one of the most critical factors affecting the process of sperm production, known as spermatogenesis. Sperm cells are produced in the testes, which are housed in the scrotum—a structure uniquely positioned outside the abdominal cavity. This external placement is no accident; it allows the testes to maintain a temperature approximately 2–3 degrees Celsius cooler than the rest of the body. This cooler environment is essential for the proper functioning of the cells responsible for sperm production. However, various factors in daily life can disrupt this delicate balance and lead to overheating of the testes, negatively impacting sperm quality.

Overheating of the testes can result from several common activities, such as wearing tight underwear, prolonged sitting, using heated car seats, or placing a laptop directly on the lap. Each of these situations raises the temperature around the scrotum, disrupting spermatogenesis. Studies have shown that even short-term increases in testicular temperature can reduce sperm count, impair motility, and increase the number of abnormally shaped sperm.

One of the primary mechanisms by which overheating affects sperm quality is **oxidative stress**. Higher temperatures promote the production of free radicals in the testes, which damage sperm DNA and cellular membranes. These damages not only reduce the sperm's ability to fertilize an egg but also increase the risk of genetic defects in offspring.

Prolonged overheating can also impair the function of Sertoli cells, which play a crucial role in nourishing and supporting developing sperm cells. Disruption of these cells' functions can lead to significant fertility problems that often require specialized medical treatment.

So, how can overheating of the testes be avoided to protect spermatogenesis? The first step is choosing the right clothing. Loose, breathable underwear made from natural materials such as cotton can help maintain the proper temperature around the scrotum. Tight briefs or pants restrict airflow and raise temperatures, negatively affecting sperm production.

Another important consideration is avoiding prolonged sitting, particularly in office jobs or during long commutes. Regularly standing up, taking short breaks, and moving around can improve blood flow and help maintain the testes' optimal temperature. If you use heated car seats, limit their use, especially on long drives.

It is also crucial to avoid placing laptops directly on your lap. Using a stand or desk not only prevents overheating but also improves posture and work comfort. Similarly, paying attention to bedroom temperatures is important—excessive heating at night can lead to overall body overheating, including the genital area.

Certain habits, such as frequent sauna visits or hot baths, can also lead to temporary reductions in sperm quality. While occasional sauna use is unlikely to have a lasting impact on fertility, regular exposure to high temperatures may require lifestyle adjustments.

In conclusion, maintaining the proper temperature of the testes is a vital component of reproductive health. Avoiding factors that cause overheating, such as tight clothing, prolonged sitting, or placing laptops on the lap, can significantly improve sperm quality and increase the likelihood of conception. Taking care of these simple aspects of daily life is an investment in reproductive health and the future of your family.

3.5. The impact of occupational hazards on reproductive health

Work plays a central role in the lives of adults, yet its potential impact on reproductive health is often underestimated. The workplace can expose individuals to various environmental risks that negatively affect sperm quality and overall male fertility. Understanding how occupational factors influence reproductive health is essential for identifying ways to mitigate these risks and safeguard long-term fertility.

One of the most prominent occupational hazards affecting reproductive health is **exposure to harmful chemicals**. Many industries, including agriculture, construction, chemical manufacturing, and even healthcare, involve regular contact with substances such as pesticides, heavy metals, solvents, and paints. These chemicals can enter the body through inhalation, skin absorption, or ingestion and accumulate in the system over time. Heavy metals like lead, cadmium, and mercury are especially damaging as they interfere with the normal functioning of the testes. Studies show that prolonged exposure to these substances can result in DNA fragmentation in sperm, reduced motility, and lower sperm counts. For example, pesticides commonly used in agriculture may disrupt hormonal balance and spermatogenesis, potentially leading to long-term fertility issues.

Another critical risk factor in certain professions is **exposure to elevated temperatures**. Men working in jobs requiring frequent or prolonged exposure to heat, such as chefs, welders, or workers in metal or glass manufacturing, are particularly vulnerable. The testes, housed in the scrotum, require a temperature 2–3 degrees Celsius lower than core body temperature for optimal spermatogenesis. Prolonged or frequent overheating in the testicular region disrupts this delicate balance, impairing sperm production. Elevated temperatures can cause a significant decline in sperm count and motility and may increase the proportion of abnormally shaped sperm. Even brief exposure to high temperatures can have a temporary but noticeable effect, emphasizing the importance of taking regular breaks and wearing protective clothing to mitigate heat exposure.

Sedentary work environments also pose a threat to male reproductive health. Jobs that involve prolonged sitting, such as those of office workers, drivers, or pilots, can restrict blood flow to the pelvic region. This lack of circulation can lead to overheating of the testes and subsequently impair sperm production. Additionally, sedentary jobs often contribute to weight gain or obesity, which is another significant risk factor for reduced sperm quality. Obesity can lead to hormonal imbalances, including reduced testosterone levels and increased estrogen, both of which negatively affect spermatogenesis. To counteract the risks associated with sedentary work, it is advisable to incorporate regular breaks for movement, stretching, or even short walks throughout the workday.

Workplace stress is another pervasive factor influencing male fertility. Chronic stress elevates levels of cortisol, a hormone that, when present in excess, suppresses testosterone production. Reduced testosterone levels can directly impact sperm production, leading to lower sperm counts, reduced motility, and decreased fertilization potential. In addition to physical effects, stress often results in psychological challenges such as reduced libido or sexual dysfunction, further complicating fertility issues. Professions with high demands, tight deadlines, or irregular hours—such as those in healthcare, emergency services, or finance—are particularly prone to causing chronic stress. Learning stress management techniques, such as mindfulness, meditation, or physical exercise, can significantly reduce its impact.

Exposure to electromagnetic radiation (EMR) is another occupational hazard that has gained attention in recent years. Workers in fields such as telecommunications, radiology, and power generation are often exposed to higher levels of EMR than the general population. While the long-term effects of EMR on sperm quality are still being studied, early evidence suggests that prolonged exposure may lead to DNA damage in sperm, reduced motility, and lower sperm viability. Taking precautions, such as following safety guidelines, maintaining a safe distance from radiation sources, and using protective equipment, can help minimize risks.

Occupational hazards are not limited to physical exposures. The demands of shift work, particularly night shifts, can disrupt the body's circadian rhythm and lead to hormonal imbalances. Sleep deprivation or irregular sleep patterns, common among shift workers, can lower testosterone levels and impair spermatogenesis. Professions in healthcare, transportation, or hospitality often require irregular schedules, making it essential to prioritize sleep hygiene and adopt strategies to maintain a consistent sleep routine wherever possible.

In addition to the direct occupational risks, lifestyle factors influenced by the workplace also play a role. For instance, jobs with high social pressures or networking demands may lead to increased consumption of alcohol or tobacco, both of which are known to harm sperm quality. High alcohol consumption can reduce testosterone levels and lead to the production of defective sperm, while smoking introduces harmful chemicals such as nicotine and cadmium, which damage sperm DNA and impair motility. Addressing these lifestyle factors by adopting healthier habits can mitigate their cumulative effects.

Mitigating occupational risks to reproductive health involves proactive measures. Employers and employees alike should prioritize health and safety practices. Workers in high-risk industries should use appropriate personal protective equipment, such as gloves, masks, or heat-resistant clothing, to minimize exposure to harmful substances and temperatures. Regular medical check-ups, including hormonal assessments and semen analysis, are crucial for detecting early signs of reproductive health issues. For sedentary workers, incorporating physical activity into daily routines and maintaining a healthy weight can significantly improve sperm quality.

Furthermore, raising awareness about the potential risks and encouraging open communication between employees and employers can foster a safer work environment. Policies promoting regular breaks, ergonomic workstations, and mental health support can help reduce both physical and psychological stressors in the workplace. Employees should feel empowered to seek adjustments or accommodations that support their well-being, particularly in high-stress or high-risk jobs.

In conclusion, the workplace can significantly influence male reproductive health, with factors such as chemical exposure, high temperatures, sedentary lifestyles, stress, and radiation playing major roles. Recognizing these risks and adopting protective measures can help maintain sperm quality and overall fertility. By combining workplace safety practices with a commitment to healthy lifestyle choices, men can safeguard their reproductive health and improve their chances of conceiving healthy offspring.

3.6. How to protect yourself from environmental risks

The environment plays a significant role in male reproductive health, and growing levels of pollution and industrialization have brought this issue into sharper focus. Daily exposure to harmful factors such as air pollution, heavy metals, pesticides, electromagnetic radiation, and chemicals in household products can severely impact sperm quality and fertility. However, there are effective ways to protect against these risks, reduce their effects, and support reproductive health.

The first step in safeguarding reproductive health is **awareness and identification of risks**. Understanding which substances and factors are harmful allows for targeted preventive measures. For instance, avoiding living near industrial plants or busy highways can reduce exposure to air pollution. Installing air purifiers at home further improves the quality of the air you breathe, reducing the inhalation of fine particulate matter and other pollutants.

A **nutritious diet** is another critical defense against environmental toxins. Consuming foods rich in antioxidants, such as vitamin C, vitamin E, selenium, and carotenoids, helps neutralize free radicals, which are a major cause of sperm DNA damage. Vegetables, fruits, nuts, and fish high in omega-3 fatty acids provide powerful support for the body's natural defenses against environmental harm. Avoiding processed foods, which may contain harmful additives, is equally important for minimizing exposure to toxins.

Limiting exposure to toxic chemicals is also essential. Everyday items such as cleaning agents, cosmetics, and paints often contain volatile organic compounds (VOCs), which can enter the body and contribute to oxidative stress. Choosing eco-friendly products free from harmful chemicals significantly reduces this exposure. Similarly, avoiding plastics containing bisphenol A (BPA) and phthalates by opting for alternatives like glass or stainless steel helps limit contact with endocrine disruptors.

Protecting against heavy metals, such as lead, cadmium, and mercury, requires awareness of their sources. Drinking filtered water and avoiding fish with high mercury content, like swordfish and certain types of tuna, can significantly reduce the accumulation of these metals in the body. Regular medical check-ups to monitor heavy metal levels can help identify and address potential problems early.

Electromagnetic radiation (EMF) emitted by electronic devices like smartphones, Wi-Fi routers, and laptops is another area of concern for reproductive health. **Minimizing direct contact with such devices** by using hands-free kits, keeping phones away from trouser pockets, and turning off wireless devices at night can help reduce long-term radiation exposure.

Regular breaks from prolonged sitting, especially for office workers, are equally important. A sedentary lifestyle can restrict blood flow in the pelvic area, potentially causing testicular overheating. Incorporating regular walks, stretches, and physical activity into your daily routine helps improve circulation and supports reproductive health.

Another critical aspect is **maintaining good sleep hygiene and ensuring adequate rest**. The body's natural detoxification processes are most effective during sleep when the immune and regenerative systems are most active. Adopting consistent sleep routines, avoiding blue light exposure before bed, and creating an optimal sleeping environment (dark, quiet, and cool) can enhance the body's ability to repair and protect itself from environmental stressors.

Finally, **regular health monitoring** is essential for proactive protection. Visiting specialists, conducting hormonal tests, and analyzing sperm quality allow for early detection of problems and timely intervention. Being aware of your reproductive health status empowers you to control factors that influence sperm quality and overall fertility.

Protecting against environmental risks requires conscious choices and daily efforts, but the benefits are immense. Prioritizing reproductive health not only improves fertility but also enhances overall well-being and quality of life.

Chapter 4:
Supplementation and Dietary Support

Nutrition is the cornerstone of our health, and its impact on the male reproductive system cannot be overstated. Today's diet, often centered around highly processed foods and lacking in essential nutrients, can significantly reduce sperm quality. In recent years, increasing attention has been given to the role of supplementation and conscious dietary support in improving reproductive health.

The production of healthy sperm is a process that requires adequate levels of nutrients such as vitamins, minerals, antioxidants, and fatty acids. These micronutrients support sperm motility, morphology, and viability, while deficiencies can lead to decreased sperm quality. Key vitamins, such as Vitamin C and E, act as powerful antioxidants, protecting sperm from oxidative damage. Meanwhile, minerals like zinc and selenium play crucial roles in regulating testosterone production and supporting proper spermatogenesis.

Modern lifestyles often do not favor adequate nutrient intake. Stress, lack of time for preparing nutritious meals, and the low quality of readily available food can result in deficiencies. In such cases, supplementation becomes a valuable tool to support the body's regeneration processes and the production of healthy sperm.

Antioxidants are a particular group of nutrients deserving attention in the context of sperm health. Sperm cells are especially sensitive to free radicals, which can damage their DNA and reduce fertilization potential. Regular consumption of antioxidant-rich foods, such as berries, leafy greens, and nuts, alongside appropriate supplementation, can significantly enhance sperm quality.

Omega-3 fatty acids are another essential component in reproductive health. Omega-3s support the structure of sperm cell membranes, improving their motility and fertilization capacity. Incorporating fatty fish like salmon or mackerel, as well as plant-based oils such as flaxseed oil, into your diet is a straightforward way to enhance sperm quality.

Chapter 4 of this book focuses on the practical aspects of supplementation and conscious dietary support. You'll learn which vitamins and minerals are essential for sperm health, how to select the right supplements, and what to consider when choosing them. We'll also discuss natural methods of dietary support, including herbs and plant-based products that can enhance reproductive health safely and effectively. Nutritional awareness is a powerful tool that empowers men to take control of their health and implement changes that deliver real results.

4.1. Essential vitamins and minerals for sperm quality

Vitamins and minerals play a fundamental role in maintaining overall health, and their importance for sperm quality and male reproductive health is especially critical. The process of spermatogenesis, or sperm production, relies heavily on the body's access to essential nutrients that support both the quality and quantity of sperm produced. Deficiencies in these nutrients can result in reduced sperm motility, DNA damage, and even fertility issues. Understanding which vitamins and minerals are essential for reproductive health can help men make informed decisions to optimize their fertility.

One of the most important nutrients for sperm health is **vitamin C**, renowned for its powerful antioxidant properties. Vitamin C helps neutralize free radicals, which can damage sperm DNA and impair motility. Research has shown that regular intake of vitamin C can improve sperm motility and reduce the proportion of abnormally shaped sperm. Good sources of vitamin C include citrus fruits, bell peppers, kiwi, and broccoli.

Vitamin E, often referred to as the "fertility vitamin," also plays a crucial role in protecting sperm from oxidative stress. Acting as a potent antioxidant, vitamin E safeguards the cell membranes of sperm against damage caused by free radicals. Consuming adequate amounts of vitamin E has been shown to enhance sperm motility and improve their ability to fertilize an egg. Vitamin E is found in nuts, almonds, sunflower seeds, and plant-based oils like olive oil and canola oil.

Zinc is another critical mineral for male reproductive health. It supports testosterone production, which is essential for spermatogenesis. Low zinc levels can lead to a reduction in sperm count and motility. Zinc also enhances sperm quality by stabilizing DNA and reducing the likelihood of damage. Rich sources of zinc include oysters, meat, pumpkin seeds, nuts, and whole grains.

Another essential nutrient is **selenium**, which plays a vital role in protecting sperm from oxidative stress and supporting their motility. A deficiency in selenium can lead to reduced sperm count and increased levels of DNA-damaged sperm. Selenium is abundant in Brazil nuts, fish, eggs, and whole grains.

Folic acid, often associated with women's reproductive health, is equally important for men. Adequate folic acid levels help in the production of healthy sperm and protect against DNA damage. Studies show that folic acid deficiency can increase the risk of genetic abnormalities in sperm. Leafy green vegetables like spinach, kale, and lettuce are excellent sources of this nutrient.

Magnesium and calcium also play significant roles in reproductive health. Magnesium contributes to sperm motility and supports hormonal functions, while calcium is critical for sperm activation during fertilization. Both minerals can be found in nuts, seeds, dairy products, and whole-grain foods.

To fully harness the benefits of vitamins and minerals, it is important to maintain a varied and balanced diet. Regular consumption of fresh fruits, vegetables, animal proteins, and plant-based fats ensures the body receives the necessary nutrients to support reproductive health. For individuals with nutrient deficiencies or those struggling to meet their nutritional needs through diet alone, supplementation may be a viable option. However, it is essential to consult a healthcare provider before starting any supplements to avoid the risks of overdosing or interactions with other medications.

In conclusion, vitamins and minerals play a pivotal role in maintaining male reproductive health. A diet rich in antioxidants, trace elements, and essential nutrients can significantly enhance sperm quality, boosting the chances of conceiving healthy offspring. Adopting healthy dietary habits is not only an investment in future family life but also in one's overall well-being.

4.2. Antioxidants: how they support sperm health

Antioxidants are essential in defending the body against oxidative stress, a leading factor affecting sperm quality. Oxidative stress arises when the body produces an excessive amount of free radicals—unstable molecules that can damage cells, including sperm. These free radicals attack cellular membranes, internal structures, and DNA, compromising sperm motility, count, and morphology. Over time, this damage can significantly impair male fertility, making antioxidants an indispensable ally for maintaining reproductive health.

Antioxidants act as a natural defense system, neutralizing free radicals and protecting cells from their harmful effects. In the context of male fertility, their importance cannot be overstated. Spermatogenesis, the process of sperm production in the testes, is particularly vulnerable to oxidative stress because it relies on a delicate balance of cellular conditions. Without adequate antioxidant protection, this balance is disrupted, and the production of healthy, viable sperm is jeopardized.

Vitamin C is one of the most crucial antioxidants for sperm health. Known for its potent free-radical-fighting properties, vitamin C safeguards sperm DNA and enhances overall sperm stability. Studies have shown that men with higher vitamin C intake experience improvements in sperm count, motility, and morphology. Additionally, vitamin C helps reduce sperm agglutination—a condition where sperm cells stick together, impairing their motility. Foods rich in vitamin C, such as citrus fruits, strawberries, bell peppers, kiwi, and broccoli, are excellent dietary sources for boosting this vital nutrient.

Equally important is **vitamin E**, often referred to as the "fertility vitamin." It protects sperm cell membranes from oxidative damage, ensuring their longevity and functionality. Vitamin E is particularly effective when combined with vitamin C, as the two antioxidants work synergistically to amplify their protective effects. Studies have demonstrated that vitamin E supplementation can improve sperm motility and enhance fertilization potential. Rich dietary sources of vitamin E include nuts, seeds, vegetable oils, and green leafy vegetables like spinach and kale.

Selenium, a trace mineral with powerful antioxidant properties, plays a critical role in sperm health. It supports the structural integrity of sperm and enhances their motility. Selenium also aids in preventing oxidative damage to sperm DNA, which is crucial for maintaining genetic stability. A deficiency in selenium has been linked to reduced sperm quality, including lower counts and abnormal morphology. Selenium can be obtained from foods such as Brazil nuts, fish, eggs, and whole grains.

Another key antioxidant is **glutathione**, a naturally occurring compound in the body that plays a pivotal role in detoxification and cellular protection. Glutathione is particularly effective at repairing oxidative damage and supporting the spermatogenesis process. Low levels of glutathione have been associated with poor sperm quality and decreased fertility, highlighting its importance in reproductive health. While the body produces glutathione naturally, it can also be boosted through the consumption of foods like avocados, asparagus, and spinach.

Coenzyme Q10 (CoQ10) is another potent antioxidant that directly impacts sperm health. Found in high concentrations in the mitochondria of sperm cells, CoQ10 is essential for energy production, which fuels sperm motility. It also protects sperm from oxidative stress, ensuring they remain viable during their journey to fertilize an egg. Research indicates that CoQ10 supplementation improves sperm parameters in men experiencing fertility challenges. Foods like fatty fish, organ meats, and whole grains are good dietary sources of CoQ10.

In addition to these specific antioxidants, a diet rich in a variety of antioxidant compounds is crucial for comprehensive protection. **Carotenoids**, such as beta-carotene, lutein, and zeaxanthin, are found in brightly colored fruits and vegetables like carrots, sweet potatoes, and bell peppers. These compounds support sperm integrity and reduce the risk of oxidative damage. Similarly, **polyphenols** found in foods like dark chocolate, green tea, and berries provide significant antioxidant benefits, further enhancing sperm quality.

The effectiveness of antioxidants is not solely dependent on dietary intake; avoiding behaviors and environmental factors that exacerbate oxidative stress is equally important. For instance, smoking introduces numerous harmful chemicals, including cadmium, which generates free radicals and damages sperm DNA. Quitting smoking is one of the most impactful steps men can take to protect their reproductive health. Similarly, excessive alcohol consumption can deplete the body's natural antioxidant reserves, weakening its ability to combat oxidative stress. Limiting alcohol intake supports the body's natural defenses and enhances the efficacy of dietary antioxidants.

Exposure to environmental pollutants, such as pesticides, heavy metals, and industrial chemicals, also contributes to oxidative stress. Choosing organic produce, using air purifiers, and avoiding exposure to contaminated water sources can reduce contact with these harmful substances. Additionally, avoiding high-heat environments, such as saunas or prolonged use of heated car seats, can minimize the risk of testicular overheating, which exacerbates oxidative stress.

Regular physical activity is another way to support antioxidant function in the body. Moderate exercise has been shown to enhance the body's production of endogenous antioxidants, such as glutathione, while also improving circulation and overall metabolic health. However, excessive or high-intensity exercise can have the opposite effect, increasing oxidative stress and potentially harming sperm quality. Striking a balance in physical activity is key to optimizing reproductive health.

Lastly, while a balanced diet rich in antioxidant-rich foods is ideal, supplementation may be beneficial for men with diagnosed deficiencies or specific fertility concerns. Supplements containing vitamin C, vitamin E, selenium, or CoQ10 are widely available and have been shown to improve sperm parameters in clinical studies. It is essential, however, to consult a healthcare professional before starting any supplementation regimen to ensure appropriate dosing and avoid potential side effects or interactions.

By understanding the role of antioxidants and incorporating them into a daily routine, men can significantly improve their reproductive health. These powerful compounds not only protect sperm from oxidative damage but also enhance their motility, count, and overall quality, increasing the likelihood of successful conception.

4.3. Dietary supplements: what to use and what to avoid

In today's fast-paced world, it can be challenging to provide the body with all the essential nutrients solely through diet. Dietary supplements have become a popular solution, especially when it comes to enhancing male reproductive health. They can improve sperm quality, increase sperm count, and boost motility, but the key lies in selecting the right supplements and avoiding those that may do more harm than good.

How Do Supplements Support Reproductive Health?

Dietary supplements provide concentrated doses of vitamins, minerals, and other compounds that support spermatogenesis—the process of sperm production. They help regulate hormonal functions, reduce oxidative stress, and protect sperm DNA from damage. However, their effectiveness depends on the quality of the supplements, individual health needs, and consistent use.

What Should You Use?

One of the most recommended supplements for men focusing on sperm health is **folic acid**. While primarily associated with women's health during pregnancy, folic acid plays a vital role in spermatogenesis by supporting cell division and maintaining sperm DNA stability. Studies indicate that men who take folic acid supplements have a lower risk of genetic abnormalities in their sperm.

Zinc is another essential mineral. It promotes testosterone production, which directly affects sperm quality. Research shows that men with higher zinc levels exhibit improved sperm count and motility. Quality zinc supplements often include vitamin B6 to further support hormonal processes.

Coenzyme Q10 (CoQ10) is gaining recognition for its benefits in addressing fertility challenges. Its antioxidant properties protect sperm mitochondria, which are responsible for energy production and motility. Regular CoQ10 supplementation enhances sperm's ability to reach and fertilize an egg, increasing the likelihood of conception.

Vitamins C and E are crucial for fighting oxidative stress, one of the leading causes of declining sperm quality. Vitamin C stabilizes sperm DNA, while vitamin E protects sperm cell membranes, improving longevity and functionality. Together, they create a synergistic effect that enhances their protective capabilities.

Selenium, a powerful antioxidant, supports sperm motility and DNA integrity. It is particularly beneficial for men exposed to high oxidative stress due to environmental factors. Selenium can be found in high-quality supplements and is often paired with other antioxidants for optimal results.

Omega-3 fatty acids, found in fish oil, are another critical component. Docosahexaenoic acid (DHA), a key omega-3 fatty acid, supports sperm cell membrane structure, improving flexibility and motility. Omega-3 supplementation is especially important for men with low dietary intake of fatty fish.

What Should You Avoid?

Not all supplements are safe or effective. It is essential to avoid products that lack scientific backing or contain excessive doses of vitamins and minerals. Over-supplementing with vitamins such as vitamin A can be toxic and cause more harm than good.

Herbal testosterone boosters are another controversial category. While they promise quick results, their effects are not always scientifically validated, and in some cases, they may disrupt the body's hormonal balance.

Unverified supplements purchased from unreliable online sources should also be avoided. These products may contain contaminants, and the lack of certification raises questions about their safety and efficacy.

74

How to Choose the Right Supplements?

Choosing the right supplements requires an informed approach. Look for products with clear ingredient lists, reputable manufacturers, and quality certifications. Supplements from well-known brands that comply with safety standards are the safest option.

Consulting a healthcare provider or nutritionist is crucial before starting supplementation. A professional can recommend products tailored to individual needs and help avoid potential interactions with other medications.

Consistent use of high-quality supplements, combined with a balanced diet, can significantly enhance sperm quality and support reproductive health.

4.4. The role of omega-3 fatty acids in reproductive wellness

Omega-3 fatty acids are among the most well-known and widely praised nutrients for overall health, but their significance for male reproductive health is equally profound. As essential polyunsaturated fatty acids, omega-3s play a critical role in many bodily functions, and their impact on sperm quality and health has become a focus of increasing attention among researchers and healthcare professionals. Let's explore why omega-3 fatty acids are so vital for reproductive health and how they can be effectively incorporated into a daily routine.

Omega-3 fatty acids come in several forms, but **docosahexaenoic acid (DHA)** and **eicosapentaenoic acid (EPA)** are particularly important for male fertility. DHA is a structural component of cell membranes, ensuring their fluidity and integrity. In sperm, DHA supports the structure of the membrane around the tail, or flagellum, which is essential for motility. EPA, on the other hand, offers potent anti-inflammatory and antioxidant properties, protecting sperm from oxidative stress that can damage their DNA and cellular structures.

One of the primary ways omega-3 fatty acids enhance sperm quality is by improving the **fluidity of sperm cell membranes**. Flexible membranes enable sperm to move efficiently, increasing their chances of reaching and fertilizing an egg. Studies show that men with higher levels of DHA in their bodies exhibit better sperm parameters, including higher count, improved motility, and better morphology.

Omega-3 fatty acids also play a crucial role in the body's **hormonal balance**, supporting testosterone production. Testosterone is the key hormone involved in spermatogenesis, the process of sperm production in the testes. Low testosterone levels can lead to reduced sperm count and poorer quality. Regular omega-3 intake helps maintain optimal testosterone levels, contributing to better reproductive health.

Another significant benefit of omega-3s is their ability to **reduce inflammation** in the body. Inflammatory processes in the reproductive system, such as infections or chronic inflammation, can negatively affect sperm quality. Omega-3 fatty acids act as natural anti-inflammatory agents, reducing inflammation and supporting tissue repair. This helps the body perform reproductive functions more effectively.

Fatty fish, such as salmon, mackerel, sardines, and tuna, are the richest sources of omega-3 fatty acids. For individuals who do not consume fish, omega-3 supplements like fish oil capsules or DHA and EPA-enriched products can provide an effective alternative. It is essential to choose high-quality supplements free from contaminants like heavy metals, which can negatively impact reproductive health.

For those seeking plant-based sources, options such as flaxseeds, chia seeds, and walnuts contain alpha-linolenic acid (ALA), a precursor to DHA and EPA. While the body can convert ALA into active forms, the conversion rate is limited, making direct consumption of DHA and EPA from fish or supplements more effective for maximizing benefits.

Maintaining the right **omega-3 to omega-6 ratio** in the diet is equally important. Modern diets, rich in processed foods and vegetable oils, often provide excessive omega-6 fatty acids, which can promote inflammation when consumed disproportionately to omega-3s. Striving for a balanced ratio with a higher intake of omega-3s is essential for reproductive health and overall well-being.

Incorporating omega-3 fatty acids into a daily diet is one of the most impactful steps men can take to improve sperm health and fertility. Through their anti-inflammatory, antioxidant, and structural support for sperm cells, omega-3s are a cornerstone of a lifestyle that promotes successful conception.

4.5. Herbs and natural remedies for fertility support

Herbs and natural remedies have been used for centuries in traditional medicine to enhance reproductive health and support fertility. Modern research increasingly validates their effectiveness, making them a popular addition to strategies aimed at improving sperm quality and overall reproductive wellness. Plant-based substances, grounded in traditional wisdom and supported by contemporary scientific studies, offer valuable support for men facing fertility challenges.

One of the most renowned herbs for fertility enhancement is **ginseng (Panax ginseng)**, often referred to as the "root of life." Ginseng is known for its adaptogenic properties, meaning it helps the body better manage stress. Stress is a significant factor that negatively impacts reproductive health, and regular use of ginseng can mitigate its effects. Additionally, ginseng has been shown to improve testosterone levels and enhance sperm count and motility.

Another highly regarded herb is **maca (Lepidium meyenii)**, a plant native to the Andes, celebrated for its ability to boost energy and libido. Studies have demonstrated that maca can also support spermatogenesis by improving sperm quality, including increased count and motility. Consuming powdered maca root or supplements derived from it can yield noticeable benefits for reproductive health.

Ashwagandha (Withania somnifera), also known as Indian ginseng, is another adaptogenic herb with fertility-enhancing properties. Ashwagandha reduces cortisol levels, the stress hormone that can disrupt hormonal balance in the body. It also promotes testosterone production, which in turn improves sperm quality and increases the likelihood of successful conception.

Tribulus terrestris, commonly known as puncture vine, is often used to boost testosterone levels and improve libido. While its hormonal effects are not fully understood, evidence suggests that it can enhance sperm quality and support the health of the reproductive system. Tribulus is available in capsule, powder, or extract form and is a popular ingredient in fertility supplements.

Although not an herb, **zinc**, a natural mineral, is frequently included in fertility therapies. Zinc supports testosterone production and healthy spermatogenesis while protecting sperm DNA from damage. Herbal blends often include zinc as a key component for reproductive health.

Fenugreek (Trigonella foenum-graecum) is another herb that may benefit men's reproductive health. Known for its ability to regulate blood sugar levels, fenugreek also supports testosterone production and improves sperm parameters. It is available in seed form, teas, or supplements.

Natural fertility remedies extend beyond herbs to include bee products such as **pollen** and **propolis**. Bee pollen is rich in antioxidants, vitamins, and minerals that enhance sperm quality. Propolis, on the other hand, has anti-inflammatory properties and supports the body's overall immunity, which indirectly contributes to reproductive health.

It is essential to recognize that while herbs and natural remedies can be beneficial, their use must be carefully considered. Choosing high-quality products from reputable manufacturers is critical, as uncontrolled dosages or contaminated preparations can do more harm than good. Consulting a healthcare professional or a specialist in natural medicine before starting any herbal regimen ensures that the chosen remedy is safe and tailored to individual needs.

4.6. How to tailor supplementation to your needs

Choosing the right supplements is a critical step in maintaining male reproductive health. Each body has unique requirements shaped by genetics, lifestyle, diet, and underlying health conditions. Selecting supplements that support sperm quality and fertility requires a thoughtful approach grounded in scientific knowledge and individual needs, avoiding a one-size-fits-all strategy.

Assessing Your Body's Needs

The first step in tailoring supplementation is evaluating your current health status. It is essential to identify specific issues that may affect sperm quality, such as low sperm count, poor motility, hormonal imbalances, or oxidative stress. Laboratory tests, including semen analysis, testosterone levels, and nutrient assessments for zinc or selenium, can provide valuable insights into potential deficiencies.

Adapting Supplementation to Your Lifestyle

Lifestyle plays a significant role in reproductive health, and supplementation should align with daily habits. For example, individuals exposed to high levels of stress may benefit from adaptogens like ashwagandha, which help the body manage tension. Men with sedentary lifestyles, often at higher risk of oxidative stress, might consider supplements rich in antioxidants such as vitamin C, vitamin E, or coenzyme Q10.

Addressing Specific Dietary Needs

Not all men can meet their nutritional requirements through diet alone. Those who do not consume fish may lack omega-3 fatty acids, which are critical for sperm quality. In such cases, supplementing with DHA and EPA from fish oil or plant-based alternatives is essential. Similarly, individuals following plant-based diets may need additional vitamin B12 or zinc, which are vital for healthy spermatogenesis.

Combining Ingredients for Greater Effectiveness

Some nutrients work synergistically, meaning their combined use enhances their benefits. For instance, vitamin E and selenium together provide more robust protection against oxidative stress than when taken separately. Similarly, zinc and vitamin B6 support testosterone production, improving sperm quality. Choosing supplements with the right combinations of ingredients can optimize their impact on reproductive health.

Avoiding Excessive Supplementation

It is crucial to avoid over-supplementation, especially with vitamins and minerals that can become toxic at high doses. For example, excessive vitamin A can damage cells, including sperm, while too much iron can burden the body and promote oxidative stress. Sticking to recommended dosages and avoiding "mega-doses" of nutrients is essential for safe and effective supplementation.

Consulting with a Healthcare Professional

Before starting supplementation, it is advisable to consult a healthcare provider, nutritionist, or specialist in natural medicine. A professional can recommend the right products based on your individual needs and suggest additional tests to identify specific health concerns.

Using Supplements Wisely

Supplements should complement, not replace, a healthy diet. A balanced diet rich in fresh vegetables, fruits, protein, and healthy fats provides the foundation upon which supplementation can build. Relying solely on supplements without addressing dietary habits may fail to deliver the desired results.

Tailoring supplementation to your body's needs is an essential part of maintaining reproductive health. An informed approach based on scientific knowledge, medical evaluations, and professional consultations can significantly enhance sperm quality and increase the likelihood of successful conception.

Chapter 5:
Health Issues and Their Impact on Sperm Quality

Male reproductive health is closely tied to overall physical well-being. We often overlook that sperm quality is not just a reflection of daily habits or environmental influences but also a mirror of what's happening inside the body. Diseases, hormonal imbalances, and even minor health neglect can significantly affect the body's ability to produce healthy sperm. Identifying and understanding these issues is a crucial step in improving sperm quality and overall health.

One of the most common health problems affecting sperm quality is hormonal imbalance. Testosterone, the primary male sex hormone, plays a vital role in spermatogenesis, the process of sperm production. Hormonal imbalances, such as low testosterone levels, can lead to reduced sperm count and motility. Symptoms like chronic fatigue, low libido, or difficulties with focus may indicate hormonal issues that require medical attention.

Infections and diseases of the genitourinary system are another major factor impacting sperm quality. Bacterial, viral, or fungal infections can damage reproductive structures, causing inflammation and impairing proper sperm production. Untreated infections can lead to more severe complications, such as blockages in the sperm ducts or permanent damage to the testes. Regular check-ups and prompt attention to unusual symptoms, such as pain, swelling, or changes in semen consistency, are essential for maintaining reproductive health.

Chronic illnesses like diabetes, hypertension, or obesity also play a significant role in male reproductive health. Diabetes can damage blood vessels and nerves, negatively impacting erections and testicular function. Obesity is associated with hormonal disruptions that can lower sperm quality. Therefore, maintaining a healthy lifestyle and managing chronic conditions are investments not only in overall health but also in fertility.

The impact of injuries and surgeries on the reproductive system should not be overlooked. Mechanical injuries to the testes, hernia surgeries, or pelvic procedures can disrupt sperm flow and lead to fertility issues. In such cases, specialist support may be necessary to identify and address the problems effectively.

Chapter 5 of this book focuses on health issues that directly affect sperm quality. We will discuss how to recognize common disorders, their symptoms, and ways to prevent them. We'll also cover when it's essential to consult a specialist and what diagnostic tests can help evaluate reproductive health. Sperm health is male health— understanding this connection allows for effective action toward improving quality of life.

5.1. Hormonal imbalances: how they affect fertility

Hormones play a fundamental role in the processes within the human body, and their balance is critical for male reproductive health. When hormone levels are disrupted, it can lead to significant fertility issues, affecting spermatogenesis, libido, and overall ability to conceive. Understanding how hormonal imbalances impact reproductive health enables men to take appropriate steps to improve their situation and increase their chances of successful conception.

Testosterone: The Cornerstone of Male Fertility

Testosterone, the primary male sex hormone, plays a pivotal role in sperm production and maintaining libido. Low testosterone levels, a condition known as hypogonadism, can result in reduced sperm count, poor motility, and diminished semen quality. Testosterone is primarily produced in the testes under the influence of luteinizing hormone (LH), which is secreted by the pituitary gland. When this process is disrupted, sperm production may slow down or cease entirely.

The Role of Other Hormones

While testosterone is essential, it is not the only hormone influencing reproductive health. Follicle-stimulating hormone (FSH) is equally important as it stimulates Sertoli cells in the testes, which are responsible for spermatogenesis. Disruptions in FSH levels can lead to abnormal sperm maturation. Additionally, excessive prolactin, a hormone responsible for lactation in women, can suppress the release of LH and FSH in men, leading to decreased testosterone levels and fertility issues.

Insulin Resistance and Its Impact on Hormones

Insulin resistance, commonly associated with metabolic syndrome, affects not only overall health but also hormonal balance. Elevated insulin levels can interfere with testosterone production and promote estrogen production, disrupting the hormonal equilibrium in men. This imbalance can result in reduced libido and erectile dysfunction, further complicating efforts to conceive.

Thyroid Disorders and Fertility

Both hypothyroidism and hyperthyroidism can significantly impact male reproductive health. Thyroid hormones regulate the body's metabolism, and their imbalance can lead to reduced sperm count and abnormal sperm morphology. Elevated thyroid hormone levels can also contribute to oxidative stress, which negatively affects semen quality.

The Influence of Stress on Reproductive Hormones

Chronic stress is one of the most common factors contributing to hormonal imbalances in men. High levels of cortisol, the stress hormone, can suppress testosterone production and disrupt the hypothalamic-pituitary-gonadal axis, which governs the production of sex hormones. Consequently, spermatogenesis slows down, resulting in reduced sperm count and quality.

Diagnosing and Treating Hormonal Imbalances

The first step in addressing hormonal imbalances is undergoing appropriate laboratory tests. Measuring levels of testosterone, LH, FSH, prolactin, and thyroid hormones can identify the issue and guide treatment. Depending on the cause of the imbalance, therapy may include hormone replacement therapy (HRT), lifestyle changes, supplementation, or pharmaceutical interventions.

The Importance of a Healthy Lifestyle

Many hormonal imbalances can be mitigated by adopting healthy habits. Regular physical activity, a balanced diet rich in essential nutrients, and stress reduction can naturally help restore hormonal balance. Limiting alcohol consumption, avoiding tobacco, and maintaining a healthy weight are particularly important, as these factors directly influence sex hormone levels.

Hormonal imbalances are a leading cause of fertility issues in men, but with proper diagnosis and treatment, it is possible to improve semen quality and increase the chances of conception. Understanding the role of hormones in reproductive health and taking action to maintain their balance is key to overcoming infertility challenges.

5.2. Infections and diseases of the genitourinary system

The health of the genitourinary system is fundamental to a man's reproductive capacity. Infections and diseases affecting this intricate system can have profound effects on sperm quality, motility, and overall fertility potential. Often, these conditions can develop silently, presenting few or no symptoms, which makes them particularly insidious. Timely diagnosis, prevention, and effective treatment are critical in maintaining optimal reproductive health.

Infections such as epididymitis, prostatitis, or urethritis are common ailments of the male reproductive system. These conditions often lead to inflammation, which is a significant contributor to oxidative stress within the body. Oxidative stress is known to damage sperm cells by attacking their membranes and DNA, compromising their functionality. Damaged sperm are less motile, less viable, and often have structural abnormalities that can drastically reduce the likelihood of successful fertilization.

Sexually transmitted infections (STIs) are among the most common causes of reproductive health issues in men. Chlamydia and gonorrhea, two prevalent STIs, have a direct and detrimental impact on fertility. Chlamydia trachomatis, the bacterium responsible for chlamydia, can cause epididymitis—an inflammation of the epididymis, where sperm mature. This condition can result in fibrosis of the seminiferous tubules, limiting the production of healthy sperm. Gonorrhea, caused by Neisseria gonorrhoeae, is another infection that can inflict significant damage on the genitourinary tract. Chronic or untreated gonorrhea can lead to scarring and blockages in the reproductive system, further compounding fertility challenges.

Viral infections, including genital herpes (caused by the herpes simplex virus, HSV) and human papillomavirus (HPV), also pose considerable risks to male reproductive health. Genital herpes may result in localized inflammation and scarring of reproductive tissues, obstructing the passage of sperm. HPV, while often asymptomatic, can negatively influence semen quality, and some strains of the virus have been linked to an increased risk of reproductive system cancers, which can further compromise fertility.

Chronic prostatitis, or inflammation of the prostate gland, is another condition with significant implications for reproductive health. The prostate produces seminal fluid, a crucial component of semen that nourishes and protects sperm. Chronic inflammation of the prostate, whether caused by bacterial infections or other factors, can reduce semen volume, impair sperm motility, and alter the chemical environment of seminal fluid, making it less supportive for sperm viability.

Fungal and parasitic infections, though less common, are also notable contributors to reproductive health problems. Candida albicans, a fungal pathogen, can cause infections that lead to localized inflammation in the reproductive tract. This inflammation disrupts the normal function of the genitourinary system, potentially reducing sperm quality. Parasites, such as Schistosoma haematobium, can cause chronic inflammation of the testes and epididymis, leading to long-term damage and reduced fertility.

The impact of these infections and diseases is not limited to physical damage. The inflammatory responses triggered by infections often result in elevated levels of white blood cells in semen, a condition known as leukocytospermia. While white blood cells are essential for fighting infections, their presence in semen generates reactive oxygen species (ROS), which exacerbate oxidative stress. This oxidative stress damages sperm cells, further reducing their viability and impairing their genetic material.

Preventing and managing infections requires a proactive approach. Regular medical check-ups with a urologist, coupled with laboratory tests such as semen analysis, microbiological cultures, and advanced molecular diagnostics like PCR (polymerase chain reaction) tests, can help identify infections at an early stage. Early diagnosis not only improves the chances of effective treatment but also minimizes the risk of long-term complications.

Treatment strategies for infections of the genitourinary system depend on the underlying cause. Bacterial infections are typically managed with targeted antibiotics, while antiviral medications are used for viral infections like genital herpes. Antifungal treatments are effective against Candida infections, and antiparasitic drugs are prescribed for parasitic infestations. In chronic conditions like prostatitis, a combination of medications, lifestyle changes, and, in some cases, physical therapy may be required to alleviate symptoms and restore function.

Prevention remains the cornerstone of maintaining genitourinary health. Practicing good hygiene, particularly in intimate areas, helps reduce the risk of bacterial and fungal infections. Using protection during sexual activity, such as condoms, significantly lowers the chances of contracting STIs. Additionally, limiting the number of sexual partners and undergoing regular screenings for STIs are essential preventive measures.

Vaccination also plays a vital role in preventing infections that impact reproductive health. The HPV vaccine, for example, is highly effective in protecting against strains of the virus that are linked to cancers and other reproductive issues. While commonly associated with women's health, the HPV vaccine is equally beneficial for men, providing protection against genital warts and reducing the risk of transmission to sexual partners.

A healthy lifestyle further enhances the body's natural defenses against infections. A diet rich in vitamins, minerals, and antioxidants supports immune function, while regular physical activity promotes circulation and overall health. Adequate sleep and stress management are also crucial, as chronic stress can weaken the immune system, making the body more susceptible to infections.

Limiting the use of substances like alcohol and tobacco is another critical factor in reducing infection risks. Both substances can impair immune function and contribute to systemic inflammation, making the body less capable of fighting off infections. For smokers, quitting is particularly important, as tobacco use has been linked to an increased risk of genitourinary infections and poorer semen quality.

Infections and diseases of the genitourinary system are a significant but often overlooked aspect of male reproductive health. By understanding the risks, taking preventive measures, and seeking timely medical care, men can protect their fertility and ensure optimal reproductive health.

5.3. Chronic illnesses and their impact on sperm quality

Chronic illnesses have a profound impact on overall health, and their effects on male reproductive health are often underestimated. Metabolic disorders, cardiovascular diseases, and chronic inflammatory conditions can negatively influence sperm quality, motility, and the chances of successful conception. Understanding the mechanisms through which chronic illnesses affect fertility enables men to adopt appropriate treatment and prevention strategies.

One of the most common chronic conditions impacting sperm quality is **type 2 diabetes**. Elevated blood sugar levels damage blood vessels and nerves, which can lead to erectile dysfunction and reduced semen quality. Diabetes also disrupts spermatogenesis, resulting in decreased sperm count and impaired motility. Furthermore, high glucose levels contribute to oxidative stress, which damages sperm at the molecular level, reducing their ability to fertilize an egg.

Obesity, often associated with diabetes and metabolic syndrome, is another significant factor affecting male fertility. Adipose tissue is an active metabolic organ that produces hormones and cytokines, disrupting the hormonal balance in the body. Excess body fat leads to reduced testosterone levels and increased estrogen production, directly impairing spermatogenesis. Additionally, obesity can cause testicular overheating, further reducing sperm quality.

Cardiovascular diseases, such as hypertension and atherosclerosis, also impact reproductive health. Damage to blood vessels and impaired circulation affect the testes' ability to produce sperm and the functionality of reproductive organs. Atherosclerosis can reduce blood flow to the testes, negatively influencing spermatogenesis and semen quality.

Chronic inflammatory conditions, such as rheumatoid arthritis or autoimmune diseases, also affect fertility. These conditions are associated with elevated levels of pro-inflammatory cytokines, which can disrupt hormonal balance and damage sperm. Moreover, medications used to treat autoimmune diseases, such as corticosteroids, can suppress spermatogenesis.

Kidney and liver diseases play an essential role in the metabolism of sex hormones. Chronic kidney disease is associated with reduced testosterone levels and sexual dysfunction, which in turn affect sperm quality. Liver diseases, such as cirrhosis, can lead to increased estrogen levels in men, negatively affecting hormonal balance and fertility.

Depression and chronic stress are also significant factors impacting reproductive health. Mental health disorders increase cortisol levels, the stress hormone, which reduces testosterone production and hampers spermatogenesis. Additionally, medications used to treat depression, such as selective serotonin reuptake inhibitors (SSRIs), may affect semen quality by reducing sperm count and motility.

Lifestyle interventions play a crucial role in managing chronic illnesses and mitigating their effects on fertility. Adopting healthy habits, such as regular physical activity, a balanced diet rich in nutrients, and avoiding alcohol and tobacco, can help minimize the adverse impact of chronic diseases on sperm quality. Monitoring health and undergoing regular medical check-ups also enable early detection of problems and effective treatment.

Understanding the relationship between chronic illnesses and male fertility is essential for improving reproductive health. Through proper diagnosis, treatment, and lifestyle changes, men can significantly enhance sperm quality and increase their chances of successful conception.

5.4. Obesity and overweight as barriers to fertility

Obesity and overweight are among the most significant health challenges of modern society. While their impact on general health is well-documented, their effects on male reproductive health receive less attention. Excess body fat not only increases the risk of metabolic disorders, cardiovascular diseases, and cancers but also leads to substantial disruptions in the functioning of the reproductive system. Obesity and overweight can influence sperm quality, hormonal balance, and other critical aspects of male fertility.

One of the most direct consequences of being overweight or obese is hormonal imbalance. Adipose tissue acts as an active endocrine organ, producing hormones and cytokines that affect the entire body. Excess fat tissue leads to reduced testosterone levels—a key hormone responsible for spermatogenesis. At the same time, estrogen production increases, disrupting reproductive processes by inhibiting sperm production and reducing sperm quality. These hormonal imbalances are particularly pronounced in men with abdominal obesity, where visceral fat is metabolically active and contributes significantly to hormonal disruption.

Obesity is also linked to testicular overheating, which directly impacts spermatogenesis. Proper sperm production requires a temperature lower than the body's core temperature, which is why the testes are located outside the abdominal cavity. Excess fat around the thighs and lower abdomen increases insulation, raising the temperature in the scrotum. Studies show that obese men have lower sperm counts and a higher proportion of structurally abnormal sperm.

Overweight and obesity negatively affect metabolism, often leading to insulin resistance and metabolic syndrome. Both conditions are associated with elevated insulin and leptin levels, which interfere with testicular function. Insulin resistance disrupts hormonal signaling in the body, exacerbating issues related to sperm production and quality. Additionally, metabolic syndrome is linked to chronic inflammation, which can damage sperm DNA.

Long-term obesity also increases the risk of developing other conditions that further impair reproductive health. For instance, obese men are more likely to suffer from sleep apnea, which reduces blood oxygen levels, leading to chronic fatigue and decreased libido. Obesity also raises the risk of cardiovascular problems, affecting blood flow to the reproductive organs, potentially resulting in erectile dysfunction.

Lifestyle changes are among the most effective ways to improve reproductive health in men with overweight and obesity. A balanced diet rich in fresh vegetables, fruits, whole grains, and healthy fats can help reduce body fat and restore hormonal balance. Regular physical activity, including both aerobic and resistance exercises, supports metabolism, improves insulin sensitivity, and reduces inflammation in the body.

Obesity and overweight are significant reproductive barriers, but they are reversible. Conscious efforts to adopt a healthier lifestyle, combined with medical and psychological support, can greatly improve sperm quality, restore hormonal balance, and increase the chances of conception. Understanding the connection between excess weight and reproductive health is key to making informed decisions and protecting fertility.

5.5. The effects of surgeries and injuries on sperm health

Male reproductive health can be significantly compromised by surgeries and injuries that affect the functionality of the reproductive system. While modern medicine provides numerous diagnostic and treatment options, understanding the potential effects of surgical interventions and mechanical trauma on sperm quality is crucial for making informed health decisions.

Surgeries in the abdominal and pelvic regions, particularly those involving the testes, prostate, or bladder, can damage anatomical structures essential for sperm production and transport. One common consequence of such procedures is scarring, which can block the vas deferens and prevent sperm from reaching the ejaculate. In some cases, nerve damage during surgery may impair the ejaculation mechanism, leading to retrograde ejaculation, where semen flows into the bladder instead of exiting the body.

Hernia repair surgeries, though widely performed, can affect reproductive health, particularly if structures within the spermatic cord are inadvertently damaged. Similarly, vasectomy, considered a safe contraceptive method, is a permanent procedure that blocks sperm from entering the semen. Even with attempts to surgically reverse a vasectomy, the success rate is not always guaranteed.

Testicular injuries are another significant factor affecting sperm quality. The testes, located outside the body in the scrotum, are especially vulnerable to trauma from falls, impacts, or accidents. Such injuries can lead to hematomas, fibrosis, and, in severe cases, the loss of function in one or both testes. Reduced testicular volume after trauma often correlates with lower testosterone levels and impaired sperm production.

Testicular torsion poses a severe threat to reproductive health. This condition occurs when a testicle twists around its own axis, cutting off blood flow. If not treated within a few hours, testicular torsion can result in tissue necrosis and necessitate removal of the affected testicle. Even with timely surgical intervention, damage from oxygen deprivation may impair sperm quality.

Spinal cord injuries also have profound effects on reproductive health. Damage to the spinal cord can disrupt the nervous functions responsible for ejaculation. Men with spinal cord injuries often experience difficulties or the inability to ejaculate, complicating natural conception. In such cases, assisted reproductive techniques, such as sperm retrieval directly from the testes, may be necessary.

Rehabilitation plays a vital role in restoring reproductive health after surgeries and injuries. Physical therapy, tailored supplementation, and hormonal support can aid in recovering the functionality of the reproductive system. However, the effectiveness of these methods depends on the extent of the damage and the time elapsed since the trauma or procedure.

Preventing injuries is as important as treating them. Using appropriate protective gear during physical activities, such as genital protectors, can significantly reduce the risk of testicular damage. Regular follow-up examinations after pelvic or abdominal surgeries help monitor potential complications and facilitate timely interventions if necessary.

Surgeries and injuries can have a profound impact on male reproductive health, but with proper diagnosis, treatment, and prevention, their negative effects can be minimized. Awareness of risks and a proactive approach to health are key to maintaining good sperm quality and fertility.

5.6. When to seek help from a specialist

Male reproductive health is often overlooked or underestimated. Many men avoid visiting a doctor, especially for fertility-related issues, which can lead to unnecessary complications. However, consulting a specialist early can prevent more serious problems, significantly improve sperm quality, and increase the chances of conceiving a child.

The first sign that it's time to consult a specialist often comes when a couple struggles to conceive after a year of regular, unprotected intercourse. Studies show that in couples facing infertility, male factors contribute to about 40% of cases. Taking prompt diagnostic steps can provide clarity about the underlying causes and lead to effective solutions.

It's also crucial to seek medical advice if symptoms suggest potential reproductive health issues. These include pain, swelling, or unusual changes in the testes, erectile dysfunction, reduced libido, unusual semen characteristics (such as low volume or altered consistency), or frequent infections of the genitourinary tract. Such symptoms might indicate infections, hormonal imbalances, or more serious conditions like varicoceles or testicular cancer.

A history of health problems, such as past injuries, surgeries involving the genitourinary system, or chronic conditions like diabetes, obesity, or autoimmune diseases, is another reason to see a specialist. All these factors can negatively affect sperm quality, and discussing them with a doctor can help develop appropriate preventative or corrective measures.

Psychological issues such as chronic stress, depression, or performance anxiety also warrant attention. Mental health has a significant impact on reproductive health, and emotional challenges can directly contribute to reduced libido, erectile dysfunction, or diminished sperm quality.

Consulting a specialist is not only about diagnostics but also an opportunity to receive guidance on building healthy habits. A doctor can recommend dietary changes, lifestyle adjustments, appropriate supplementation, or hormonal therapy. In more advanced cases, they might suggest genetic, hormonal, or semen analysis to uncover the root causes of infertility.

Visiting a specialist does not mean the situation is hopeless. Modern medicine offers numerous effective treatment options, from medication and surgical procedures to advanced assisted reproductive technologies like intrauterine insemination or in vitro fertilization. Many fertility issues can be successfully addressed through these approaches.

The key is not to delay seeking professional advice. The earlier the problem is identified, the higher the chances of effective treatment. While taking this step may feel daunting, it's important to remember that reproductive health is an integral part of overall well-being. Addressing these concerns can positively impact not just fertility but also overall quality of life.

Chapter 6:
Building Healthy Habits for the Future

Male reproductive health isn't just a matter of the "here and now"—it's an investment in the future. Building healthy habits that support sperm quality and overall well-being takes time, patience, and consistency. However, it's an effort that yields multidimensional benefits, both in the context of family planning and maintaining physical and mental fitness over the long term.

The key to success in safeguarding reproductive health is understanding that the habits you adopt today have a tangible impact on your life years, or even decades, down the line. A long-term perspective allows you to make choices that not only improve sperm quality but also enhance overall wellness. Regular physical activity, a balanced diet, avoiding harmful substances, and managing stress are foundational habits that bring benefits across all areas of life.

One of the most critical aspects of caring for the future is consistency. Establishing stable, healthy routines—such as daily exercise, consistent sleep schedules, and regular meal times—supports hormonal balance and the body's natural recovery processes. It's not about perfection—it's about persistence, which gradually leads to positive changes. Even small steps, like reducing sugar intake or adding 30 minutes of walking to your daily routine, can have a meaningful impact on health.

Education and awareness are additional pillars upon which to build a long-term health strategy. Understanding how your body works, what it needs, and how it responds to changes enables better decision-making. Regular health check-ups are a vital part of this education.

They allow potential issues to be detected early, preventing them from developing into problems that could impact reproductive health.

The importance of emotional support and communication cannot be overlooked. Reproductive health is often a topic that's avoided in conversations, but open discussions with your partner or a specialist can help you better understand your needs. Building healthy habits becomes more manageable when supported by an environment that motivates and inspires action.

Chapter 6 of this book focuses on how to develop habits that yield long-term benefits, step by step. We'll discuss how to structure your day around reproductive health, what lifestyle changes to implement, and how to overcome challenges that may arise along the way. You'll see that healthy habits are not just a responsibility but also an opportunity to improve your quality of life and enjoy everyday actions. It's a journey that starts with small steps but leads to significant outcomes.

6.1. How to maintain reproductive health throughout life

Male reproductive health is deeply interconnected with overall physical and emotional well-being, requiring consistent attention and care throughout life. While sperm quality and fertility potential may naturally decline with age, numerous strategies exist to help preserve and enhance reproductive health at every stage of life. Understanding that reproductive health is not a one-time consideration but an ongoing process is vital for achieving long-term wellness and fertility.

In adolescence and early adulthood, establishing healthy habits is crucial as they lay the foundation for future reproductive health. Regular physical activity plays a key role in maintaining a healthy weight and supporting proper hormonal balance, which is essential for spermatogenesis—the production of sperm. A balanced diet rich in whole grains, fruits, vegetables, lean proteins, and healthy fats provides the necessary nutrients for optimal sperm production. Avoiding harmful substances like tobacco, recreational drugs, and excessive alcohol consumption is particularly important during this formative stage, as these substances can have long-lasting negative effects on sperm quality.

Education about reproductive health should also begin early. Young men should be informed about the risks associated with sexually transmitted infections (STIs) and the importance of safe sexual practices. Unprotected sex or multiple partners can increase the likelihood of contracting infections such as chlamydia or gonorrhea, which can severely damage the reproductive system and reduce fertility. Learning about preventive measures, such as using condoms and seeking regular health screenings, is an important step toward protecting reproductive health.

As men enter their 30s and 40s, hormonal balance becomes a central focus of reproductive health. Testosterone levels naturally decline with age, which can lead to a reduction in sperm production, decreased libido, and overall energy levels. Regular blood tests to monitor testosterone levels, as well as other key hormones like luteinizing hormone (LH) and follicle-stimulating hormone (FSH), can provide valuable insights into hormonal health. If imbalances are detected, lifestyle changes or medical interventions, such as hormone replacement therapy, may be considered under professional guidance.

Chronic stress, which is increasingly common in modern lifestyles, poses a significant threat to reproductive health. Stress activates the body's hypothalamic-pituitary-adrenal (HPA) axis, leading to elevated levels of cortisol, a stress hormone that can suppress testosterone production and disrupt the hypothalamic-pituitary-testicular axis—a critical regulator of sperm production. Managing stress through techniques like mindfulness, meditation, yoga, or regular exercise can mitigate these effects and support hormonal equilibrium.

Environmental factors also play a significant role in male reproductive health. Exposure to air pollution, heavy metals, pesticides, and endocrine-disrupting chemicals found in plastics and personal care products can negatively impact sperm quality. Even daily habits, such as placing laptops directly on the lap, can raise scrotal temperatures and impair spermatogenesis. Men should aim to minimize exposure to harmful substances by choosing organic foods, avoiding unnecessary plastic use, and being mindful of workplace hazards, particularly in industries involving chemicals or radiation.

Physical activity remains an important aspect of reproductive health throughout life. However, moderation is key. While regular exercise supports cardiovascular health, hormonal balance, and overall well-being, overtraining or excessive physical strain can elevate cortisol levels and disrupt reproductive function. Activities like swimming, running, cycling, or yoga are excellent for promoting blood circulation and reducing oxidative stress without overburdening the body. Strength training, when done in moderation, can also enhance testosterone production.

Diet continues to be a cornerstone of reproductive health as men age. Antioxidant-rich foods, including berries, citrus fruits, nuts, seeds, and green leafy vegetables, combat oxidative stress—a major contributor to sperm damage. Key nutrients like zinc, selenium, and vitamins C and E are particularly beneficial for maintaining sperm health and motility. Omega-3 fatty acids, found in fatty fish, flaxseeds, and walnuts, are known to improve sperm membrane fluidity, supporting overall sperm functionality. Avoiding processed foods, trans fats, and excessive sugar is equally important, as these can contribute to weight gain and hormonal imbalances.

Regular health screenings are another essential component of lifelong reproductive health. Men should schedule periodic visits to a urologist or reproductive specialist to monitor sperm quality, hormone levels, and overall reproductive system health. Semen analysis, which assesses parameters like sperm count, motility, and morphology, can provide valuable insights into fertility status. Additionally, self-examinations of the testes are critical for early detection of abnormalities such as lumps, swelling, or pain, which could indicate conditions like varicoceles or testicular cancer.

Preventative care extends to addressing underlying health conditions that may impact reproductive health. Chronic illnesses such as diabetes, hypertension, or obesity can adversely affect sperm quality and overall fertility. Managing these conditions through lifestyle changes, medication, or both can significantly improve reproductive outcomes. For example, maintaining a healthy weight reduces the risk of hormonal imbalances caused by excess adipose tissue, which produces estrogen and suppresses testosterone.

Emotional well-being is also an integral part of reproductive health. Mental health challenges, such as anxiety or depression, can interfere with sexual function and reduce fertility. Seeking support from a therapist or counselor, practicing relaxation techniques, and building a strong social support network can help men navigate emotional challenges and maintain a healthy outlook on life and reproduction.

By adopting a proactive approach to reproductive health, men can preserve their fertility and overall well-being throughout their lives. Regular self-care, awareness of potential risks, and a commitment to healthy habits are fundamental to maintaining optimal reproductive function. Taking control of reproductive health is not only about preparing for parenthood but also about enhancing quality of life and promoting long-term wellness.

6.2. Family planning: sperm health and a man's age

Family planning is one of the most significant challenges couples face at different stages of life. While much focus is placed on women's reproductive health, the role of men in conception and the impact of their age on sperm quality often go overlooked. However, research clearly shows that a man's age can substantially affect sperm quality, fertility potential, and even the health of his offspring.

Unlike women, who are born with a finite number of eggs, men produce sperm throughout their lives. Nevertheless, the process of spermatogenesis gradually declines with age. Around the age of 35, noticeable changes in sperm parameters begin to emerge, including a reduction in sperm count, motility, and morphology. As men age, there is also an increased risk of DNA damage in sperm, which can lead to difficulties in conception, a higher incidence of miscarriages in their partners, and an elevated risk of genetic disorders in their children.

The decline in sperm quality with age is linked to several biological factors. One key factor is the natural decrease in testosterone levels, a hormone essential for spermatogenesis. Hormonal changes associated with aging can also reduce semen volume and the number of progressively motile sperm. Additionally, the body's ability to repair DNA damage in sperm diminishes over time, increasing the likelihood of genetic mutations.

A man's overall health plays a critical role in maintaining sperm quality as he ages. Chronic conditions such as diabetes, hypertension, and obesity, which are more prevalent in middle and later life, can significantly impair sperm quality. These factors contribute to hormonal imbalances, inflammation, and vascular damage, all of which negatively affect the reproductive system's functionality.

Lifestyle choices also have a profound impact on sperm health in later years. Smoking, excessive alcohol consumption, and a sedentary lifestyle can accelerate the decline in sperm quality. Men planning to have children later in life should prioritize a healthy lifestyle, including a balanced diet rich in antioxidants that protect sperm from damage.

Exposure to harmful chemicals and environmental toxins is another critical consideration for family planning at an older age. Working in hazardous environments, exposure to pesticides or toxic substances, and prolonged exposure to high temperatures can significantly decrease sperm quality. Wherever possible, it is advisable to minimize such exposures or use protective measures.

Regular health screenings, including semen analysis, hormone level assessments, and genetic testing, are particularly recommended for middle-aged men planning to conceive. These tests can help identify potential issues and guide interventions to improve sperm quality. Consulting a urologist or fertility specialist can also provide valuable insights into reproductive health and personalized recommendations for optimizing fertility.

While a man's age does influence sperm quality, it does not mean that fathering a child later in life is impossible. By adopting lifestyle changes, using appropriate supplementation, and practicing preventive care, men can significantly enhance their chances of healthy fatherhood. Understanding that sperm health is dynamic and can be influenced is crucial for making informed family planning decisions at any age.

6.3. The importance of regular medical check-ups

Regular health check-ups play a vital role in maintaining male reproductive health at every stage of life. With the growing challenges of modern living, such as stress, environmental pollution, and unhealthy habits, preventive healthcare has become more important than ever. Systematic monitoring of health not only helps identify potential problems early but also allows for effective treatment and prevention of more serious complications.

One of the most critical examinations for men is a **semen analysis**. This simple and non-invasive test provides essential information about sperm quality, including sperm count, motility, and morphology. Regular semen analysis is particularly important for men planning to conceive, as it evaluates whether sperm quality is sufficient for natural conception. If abnormalities are detected, targeted interventions can be implemented to improve semen parameters.

Another key evaluation is the **assessment of hormone levels**, including testosterone, luteinizing hormone (LH), and follicle-stimulating hormone (FSH). These hormones are central to spermatogenesis, and their imbalances can lead to reduced sperm quality, diminished libido, and other health issues. Regular hormonal testing allows for the early detection of hormonal imbalances and facilitates appropriate treatment.

An **ultrasound examination of the testes** is another essential diagnostic tool for reproductive health. Ultrasound can detect abnormalities such as varicoceles, cysts, or tumors, which may negatively affect sperm quality and overall fertility. Varicoceles, which are common, are one of the leading causes of reduced sperm quality, and early detection enables effective treatment.

Regular **blood tests** are equally important for assessing overall health and identifying factors that may impact reproductive health, such as diabetes, vitamin deficiencies, or metabolic disorders. High blood sugar levels or insulin resistance can lower sperm quality, making early diagnosis crucial for preventing complications.

Genetic testing is another step worth considering, especially for couples struggling with infertility. Certain genetic abnormalities, such as Y-chromosome microdeletions or mutations in genes responsible for spermatogenesis, can cause infertility. Early diagnosis of these issues enables targeted treatment or the use of assisted reproductive technologies.

Preventive care also includes regular visits to a **urologist**, who can assess the condition of the prostate, testes, and other genitourinary organs. Prostate issues, such as inflammation or enlargement, can directly impact sperm quality and overall comfort. A urologist can also provide guidance on maintaining a healthy lifestyle and recommend additional tests if necessary.

Regular health check-ups not only help identify potential health problems but also enable men to take an active role in managing their reproductive health. These evaluations allow for the identification of areas requiring improvement and the monitoring of progress achieved through lifestyle changes, supplementation, or medical therapies.

It's important to note that health check-ups are particularly crucial for men over the age of 35, as this is when natural declines in sperm quality associated with aging may become apparent. However, regardless of age, regular monitoring of reproductive health helps maintain optimal semen parameters and increases the chances of conceiving healthy offspring.

Caring for reproductive health is an investment in the future—for both oneself and one's family. Regular health check-ups are a simple yet highly effective way to preserve fertility and maintain overall well-being.

6.4. Talking about reproductive health with your partner

Discussing reproductive health can be challenging, especially in relationships where fertility has become a central concern. For many men, this topic is sensitive and often accompanied by fears of judgment or guilt. However, open and honest communication with your partner is a vital step toward building mutual understanding and taking actions that can improve the situation. Caring for reproductive health is a shared responsibility, and the conversation should take place in an atmosphere of trust and mutual support.

The first step in discussing reproductive health is to create a comfortable environment for the conversation. Choose a time when both partners can talk calmly, without external distractions or time pressures. Start by expressing your feelings and intentions clearly, for example: "I'd like to talk about something important that affects both of us." This approach demonstrates that the issue is not just one person's burden but a shared challenge.

Using empathetic and understanding language during the conversation is crucial. Avoiding blame or accusations is key to productive communication. For instance, instead of saying, "It's your fault we're having trouble conceiving," try, "I'd like to understand what we can do together to improve our chances of conceiving." This type of language fosters connection and shows that both partners are committed to finding solutions.

Sharing facts and knowledge about reproductive health can also be helpful. This might include information about factors that influence sperm quality, such as diet, lifestyle, or stress. If you've already undergone medical tests, discussing the results openly and inviting your partner to explore possible solutions together can be a constructive step. For many women, understanding the biology of male fertility can be an enlightening experience that fosters greater empathy and awareness.

Equally important is listening to your partner and allowing her to express her feelings and concerns. Fertility is an emotional subject for many women as well, and an open conversation can help address fears or frustrations. It's important to emphasize that there is no single "culprit" when it comes to fertility challenges—it's a shared issue that requires cooperation from both sides.

Talking about reproductive health can also be an opportunity to discuss shared goals and plans for the future. This might involve decisions about lifestyle changes, such as adopting a healthier diet, increasing physical activity, or reducing substance use. Your partner can also be a valuable source of support in monitoring these changes and encouraging you to maintain them. Working together strengthens the bond and shows that both partners are invested in achieving a shared goal.

Don't hesitate to seek professional help. A joint visit to a urologist, andrologist, or fertility specialist can be a step that reduces tension and helps both partners better understand the situation. A doctor can also serve as a mediator in discussions about reproductive health, providing professional insights and guidance.

Discussing reproductive health not only helps address fertility challenges but also strengthens the relationship. Open communication builds trust, enables partners to better understand each other, and fosters collaborative decision-making that can positively impact their lives. The key is an approach rooted in understanding, empathy, and a willingness to work together—this is the foundation for successfully navigating health challenges in a relationship.

6.5. Education and awareness: promoting healthy habits within the family

Education and health awareness are not only tools for improving one's lifestyle but also a way to instill healthy habits within the family. Shared efforts, knowledge exchange, and implementing changes in daily routines are essential to promoting long-term reproductive and overall health among family members. Building these habits not only supports fertility but also strengthens family bonds and prepares future generations to make informed health decisions.

The first step in promoting healthy habits in the family is open communication about reproductive health and its importance. This topic may seem challenging, especially in cultures where fertility and reproductive health are considered taboo. However, education begins with conversation. Parents can approach this naturally by explaining to younger family members how a healthy lifestyle positively impacts the body, including the reproductive system. These discussions don't need to be overly detailed but should emphasize the role of health in achieving life goals, such as starting a family.

It's equally important that education is grounded in reliable knowledge. In the digital age, access to information is easier than ever, but not all sources are trustworthy. Parents and caregivers should rely on scientific literature, expert-written guides, and consultations with doctors and reproductive health specialists. This knowledge can then be shared in simple, understandable ways tailored to the age and needs of family members.

Shaping healthy habits in the family also requires practical actions. Regular family meals, prepared with a focus on nutritious eating, can be an opportunity to learn about foods that promote reproductive health. For instance, cooking meals rich in zinc, selenium, or antioxidants not only introduces beneficial nutrients into the diet but also teaches younger generations the value of such ingredients and their health benefits.

Equally important is incorporating physical activity into family life. Activities like walks, bike rides, team sports, or other forms of exercise can improve physical health while providing opportunities for quality time together. Physical activity supports cardiovascular health, which is essential for the proper functioning of the reproductive system. Moreover, shared exercises strengthen family bonds and demonstrate the importance of perseverance in achieving health goals.

Promoting healthy habits also involves educating about avoiding harmful factors, such as smoking, excessive alcohol consumption, or exposure to toxic substances. Parents can act as role models, showing their children how to avoid these risks and the benefits of maintaining a healthy lifestyle. The example set by older family members is one of the most effective ways to establish positive behavior patterns in children and adolescents.

Sex education plays a crucial role in building health awareness. Knowledge about the functioning of the reproductive system, fertility, and protection against sexually transmitted infections (STIs) forms the foundation of reproductive health. This education should be open and age-appropriate, fostering curiosity and understanding rather than shame or embarrassment.

Long-term promotion of healthy habits within the family requires consistency and commitment. Establishing schedules for regular medical check-ups, implementing small but sustainable lifestyle changes, and encouraging family members to prioritize health are actions that yield tangible benefits. A family that collectively cares for its health not only enhances its quality of life but also provides children with the tools to make responsible decisions in the future.

6.6. Small changes, big results: how to sustain healthy sperm

Caring for male reproductive health often feels like a daunting task, requiring major lifestyle overhauls or complex interventions. However, studies show that even small, consistent changes in daily habits can have a profound impact on sperm quality and overall fertility. The secret lies in making manageable adjustments that, over time, become part of a sustainable and healthy routine. These incremental steps, when maintained consistently, can yield big results.

The first area to focus on is diet. It's not necessary to adopt an entirely new meal plan overnight—starting with simple adjustments can make a noticeable difference. For example, adding a handful of nutrient-dense foods to your daily routine can have a significant impact. Walnuts and almonds, rich in omega-3 fatty acids, can improve sperm motility and membrane integrity. Similarly, increasing the consumption of leafy greens like spinach or kale provides folate, a nutrient essential for DNA synthesis and cell division, which are critical during sperm maturation. Antioxidant-rich foods such as berries, citrus fruits, and tomatoes can help reduce oxidative stress, a major factor in sperm damage.

Incorporating lean proteins, such as chicken, fish, or plant-based sources like legumes, into your diet ensures the body receives adequate amino acids for hormone production and tissue repair. Meanwhile, limiting processed foods and sugary snacks can prevent weight gain and improve hormonal balance, both of which are essential for optimal sperm health. Hydration is equally important—ensuring adequate water intake supports overall cellular function, including in reproductive cells.

Physical activity is another area where small, gradual changes can lead to significant improvements. Regular exercise boosts cardiovascular health, reduces stress, and promotes hormonal balance—all of which contribute to healthier sperm. Starting with low-impact activities, like walking or cycling, can help build a foundation for more rigorous workouts. Moderate-intensity exercise, performed consistently, enhances blood flow to the reproductive organs, ensuring an adequate supply of nutrients and oxygen for sperm production.

However, balance is key. Overtraining or engaging in high-intensity exercise without proper recovery can increase cortisol levels, the body's stress hormone, which negatively impacts testosterone production and spermatogenesis. Aiming for 30 minutes of moderate exercise, such as swimming, jogging, or yoga, most days of the week is an excellent starting point. Stretching and relaxation-focused exercises can also aid in reducing muscle tension and improving overall well-being.

Reducing exposure to harmful substances is another critical step. Smoking, excessive alcohol consumption, and recreational drug use are among the top contributors to poor sperm quality. Smoking, in particular, is associated with increased DNA fragmentation in sperm and reduced motility. For those who smoke, quitting is one of the most impactful decisions for improving reproductive health. Reducing alcohol intake to moderate levels—defined as one or two drinks a day—can help mitigate its effects on hormonal balance and sperm production.

Environmental factors also play a significant role in sperm health. Avoiding prolonged exposure to high temperatures, such as in saunas, hot tubs, or long hot showers, is essential for maintaining optimal scrotal temperature, which is crucial for spermatogenesis. Similarly, men who work in high-temperature environments or spend long hours sitting should take regular breaks to stand, stretch, and cool down. Avoid placing laptops directly on the lap, as the heat emitted can negatively impact sperm production over time.

Another overlooked but crucial factor is sleep. Quality rest supports overall hormonal health, including the production of testosterone, which plays a direct role in sperm development. Simple adjustments like setting a regular bedtime, creating a comfortable sleep environment, and minimizing exposure to blue light from electronic devices before bed can improve both the quantity and quality of sleep. Aim for at least seven to eight hours of restful sleep each night to allow the body to fully recover and regenerate.

Stress management is an integral part of reproductive health, as chronic stress can lead to elevated cortisol levels, which suppress testosterone and disrupt sperm production. Introducing stress-relief practices into daily life, such as mindfulness meditation, deep breathing exercises, or spending time in nature, can help regulate stress hormones and improve mental clarity. Even dedicating just 10 minutes a day to a relaxation technique can make a measurable difference in stress levels and overall well-being.

Supplements can also play a supporting role, especially for men with specific deficiencies. Nutrients such as zinc, selenium, and vitamins C and E are proven to support sperm health. Omega-3 fatty acids, found in supplements or fatty fish, improve sperm motility and membrane fluidity. However, it's important to consult a healthcare provider before starting any supplement regimen to ensure it aligns with individual health needs.

Consistency is the most important factor when making these changes. Small adjustments may not yield immediate results, as sperm production takes approximately three months from start to finish. However, the cumulative effects of sustained improvements in diet, exercise, sleep, and stress management can lead to significant changes over time. Healthy sperm are not only a marker of fertility but also an indicator of overall health, reflecting the body's well-being on a cellular level.

Finally, remember that maintaining healthy sperm is not just about fertility—it's about investing in long-term health and quality of life. The steps taken to improve reproductive health, such as eating nutritious foods, staying active, managing stress, and avoiding harmful substances, contribute to better physical and emotional health. These positive changes can extend beyond personal benefits, influencing family and community health by serving as a model of wellness.

By taking small, consistent steps toward healthier habits, men can significantly improve their reproductive health. These incremental changes, while manageable, lead to profound results over time, ensuring not only improved sperm quality but also enhanced overall well-being and vitality.

Conclusion

The conclusion of this journey into male reproductive health marks the beginning of a new chapter in caring for your body, mind, and future. Sperm quality, often considered a taboo topic, is a crucial indicator of a man's overall health. This book aimed not only to provide knowledge about how to improve sperm quality but also to encourage a broader perspective on health as a whole.

Each chapter explored – from understanding the mechanisms of spermatogenesis, the importance of diet and lifestyle, to the impact of environmental factors and health issues – was designed to highlight the many factors that shape reproductive health. The key takeaway from this book is that sperm quality is not fixed or unchangeable. It is a dynamic aspect of health that can be improved through conscious choices and daily actions.

Improving sperm quality doesn't require a revolution, but rather small, consistent steps. Changes in daily habits – regular meals, physical activity, stress reduction, and better recovery – lead to lasting effects. It's important to remember that caring for reproductive health is not just an investment in the ability to have children, but also in overall quality of life, improved well-being, and greater resilience to the challenges of modern life.

I would also like to emphasize the importance of education and openness about reproductive health. Too often, men avoid this topic, considering it shameful or too personal. However, open conversations with your partner, a specialist, or even friends can be crucial for understanding your needs and finding appropriate solutions. Sperm health is not just an individual matter but also a component of building relationships and trust in a partnership.

As we conclude, I encourage you to take further action. This book is just the beginning—a tool to help you better understand your body and make informed decisions. The next steps are up to you. Perhaps you'll decide to make small dietary changes, start regular health check-ups, or seek professional support. Every step, no matter how small, brings you closer to better health and a better life.

I wish you success on this journey. Remember, taking care of sperm quality is taking care of yourself—your health, your future, and your family. It's a decision that yields benefits at every stage of life.

Summary of the key principles of reproductive health

Male reproductive health is intrinsically linked to overall well-being and lifestyle choices. Although often overlooked, maintaining sperm quality and fertility is essential not only for family planning but also for long-term physical and emotional health. Understanding the key principles that influence reproductive health is the first step toward making positive changes.

First and foremost, sperm quality largely reflects daily habits. A healthy diet rich in antioxidants, zinc, selenium, and omega-3 fatty acids is fundamental to supporting spermatogenesis. Reducing the intake of processed foods, trans fats, and simple sugars helps maintain a healthy weight and hormonal balance, both of which are crucial for reproductive health.

Physical activity is another pillar of reproductive wellness. Regular, moderate exercise improves circulation, reduces stress, and enhances overall fitness. However, it's important to avoid overtraining, which can increase cortisol levels and negatively affect testosterone production and sperm development.

Equally important is avoiding harmful substances like tobacco, alcohol, and recreational drugs, which have proven detrimental effects on sperm quality. Even small changes, such as reducing alcohol consumption or quitting smoking, can lead to significant improvements in semen parameters.

Sleep and recovery are critical components of reproductive health. Consistent, restorative sleep supports hormonal balance and, in turn, reproductive function. Simple adjustments, such as reducing exposure to blue light before bedtime or establishing regular sleep schedules, can quickly yield positive results.

Stress management plays a vital role in overall health. Chronic stress disrupts hormonal balance and impacts the entire body. Incorporating relaxation techniques such as meditation, deep breathing, or walks in nature can help reduce cortisol levels and improve mental and physical well-being.

Regular health check-ups are the cornerstone of preventive care. Semen analysis, hormone level assessments, and consultations with a urologist or andrologist enable the early detection of potential issues and the implementation of appropriate treatments. Education about reproductive health and a willingness to make informed health decisions are essential for success in this area.

In conclusion, reproductive health is the result of a holistic approach to lifestyle and daily choices. Even small, gradual changes made consistently can yield significant improvements. Caring for sperm health is not only an investment in future parenthood but also in overall quality of life and long-term well-being.

Inspiration for further care and improvement of fertility

Taking care of reproductive health and fertility is not a one-time effort or decision. It's a lifelong journey that requires ongoing attention, a willingness to learn, and the ability to adapt. The growing awareness of the impact of environmental factors, lifestyle choices, and advancements in medicine on fertility inspires individuals to take proactive steps, not only to improve reproductive health but also to enhance overall quality of life.

One of the most accessible sources of inspiration is continuous education. Regularly reading articles, books, and scientific research about reproductive health helps uncover which habits and factors have the most significant impact on sperm quality and fertility. The options are nearly endless—from subscribing to medical journals to attending webinars hosted by men's health experts. Staying informed about new discoveries and technologies can provide practical tools and insights to support reproductive wellness.

Practical actions can also serve as a source of motivation. For example, introducing new, healthy recipes into your daily diet can be both beneficial for your body and enjoyable. Experimenting with dishes rich in zinc, selenium, antioxidants, and omega-3s can offer fresh culinary experiences while supporting sperm health. Joining groups or online communities that share recipes, experiences, and lifestyle tips can further fuel motivation and provide a sense of camaraderie.

Travel and connecting with nature are other inspiring ways to support health. Activities like hiking, cycling, or simply taking walks in natural settings not only reduce stress but also strengthen the body and mind. These pursuits can become a regular part of life, improving overall well-being while also contributing to reproductive health.

Another step involves developing effective stress management techniques. Practices like meditation, yoga, or deep breathing exercises not only support hormonal balance but also teach how to respond effectively to life's challenges. Attending mindfulness workshops or using mobile apps offering relaxation programs can be excellent ways to begin these practices.

Regular consultations with specialists are a cornerstone of ongoing reproductive health care. Visits with urologists, andrologists, or dietitians can provide valuable information and support for planning the next steps. Specialized testing can also offer reassurance that the efforts being made are producing the desired outcomes.

It's important to remember the role of your partner and family in this journey. Discussions about reproductive health, planning meals together, or engaging in physical activities as a team strengthen bonds and create an atmosphere of mutual understanding. Reproductive health is not a challenge to face alone—collaborative efforts often yield better results and enrich relationships.

Taking care of health and fertility is a process that demands commitment but also openness to change and inspiration drawn from everyday life. Every step—from small dietary adjustments to regular exercise and expanding your knowledge—brings you closer to the goal of not just improved fertility, but a healthier, more fulfilling life overall.

www.ingramcontent.com/pod-product-compliance
Lightning Source LLC
Chambersburg PA
CBHW071035250726

48653CB00005B/1853